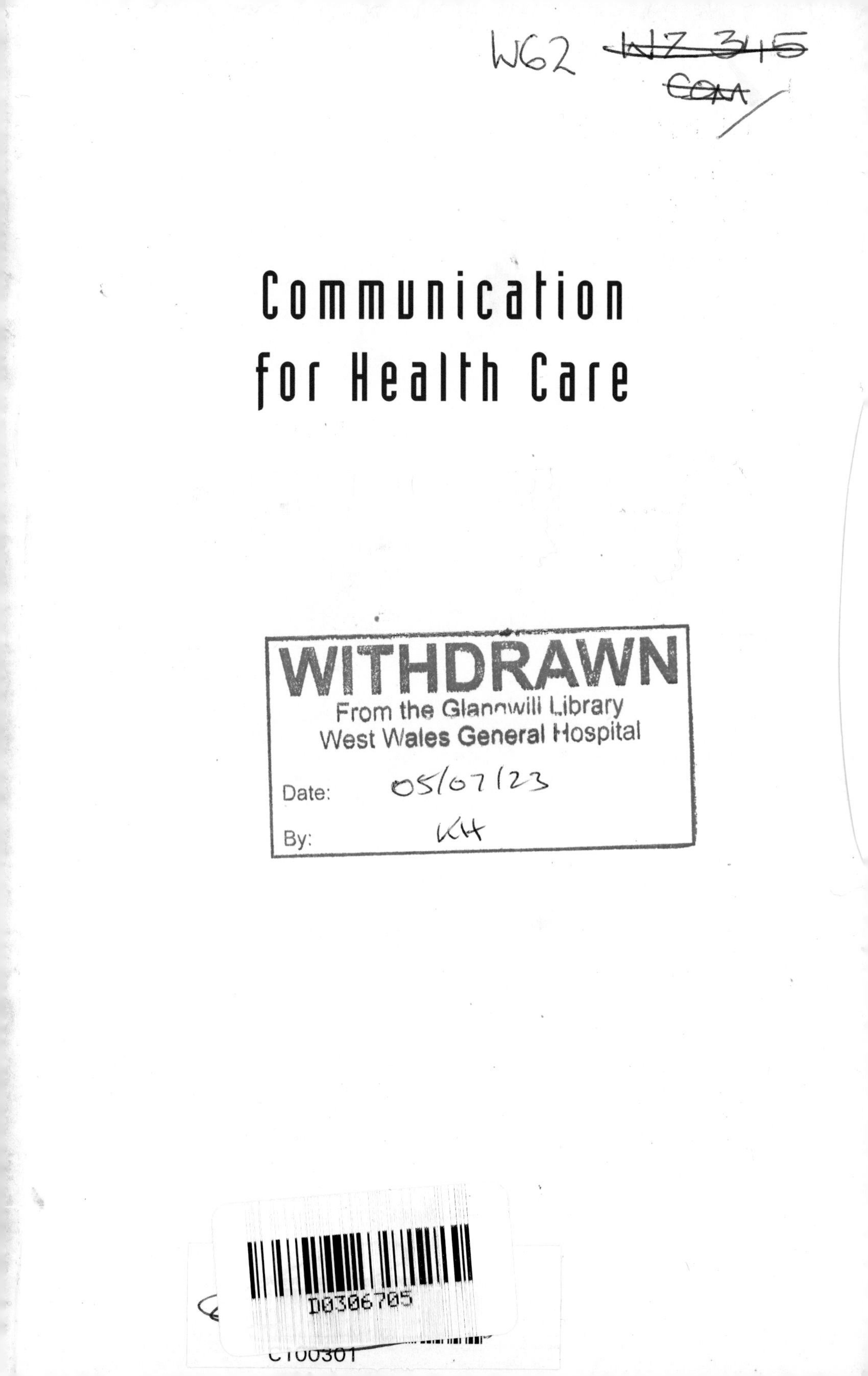

Communication for Health Care

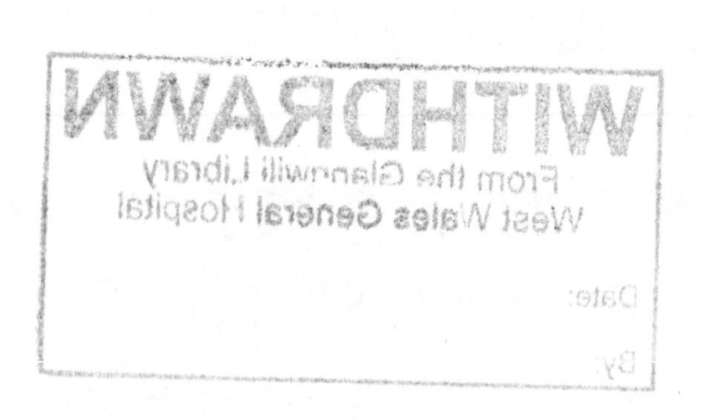

Communication for Health Care

Edited by
Catherine Berglund
and Deborah Saltman

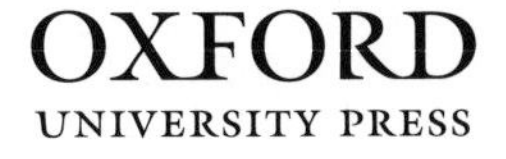

OXFORD
UNIVERSITY PRESS

253 Normanby Road, South Melbourne, Australia

Oxford University Press is a department of the University of Oxford.
It furthers the University's objective of excellence in research, scholarship, and education by publishing worldwide in

Oxford New York

Auckland Bangkok Buenos Aires Cape Town
Chennai Dar es Salaam Delhi Hong Kong Istanbul
Karachi Kolkata Kuala Lumpur Madrid Melbourne
Mexico City Mumbai Nairobi São Paulo Shanghai
Singapore Taipei Tokyo Toronto

with an associated company in Berlin

First published 2002

National Library of Australia
Cataloguing-in-Publication data:

Communication for health care.

Bibliography.
Includes index.
ISBN 0 19 551298 7.

1. Communication in medicine. 2. Medical personnel and patient.
3. Health care teams. I. Berglund, Catherine Anne. II. Saltman, Deborah.

610.696

Indexed by Russell Brooks
Text designed by Desktop Concepts Pty Ltd, Melbourne
Cover designed by Patrick Cannon
Typeset by Desktop Concepts Pty Ltd, Melbourne
Printed through Bookpac Production Services, Singapore

Contents

Tables

Figures

Contributors

Peter Baume, AO MBBS (Hons) Litt D BS FRACP FAFPHM FRACGP (Hon)
Emeritus Professor, University of New South Wales, Sydney, and
Chancellor, Australian National University, Canberra (Chapter 14)

Catherine Berglund, BSc (Psychol) PhD (Community Medicine)
Senior Lecturer in Ethics, School of Public Health and Community Medicine, University of New South Wales, Sydney (joint editor; author of Chapters 1, 8, and 15)

Alan Cartwright, B Com
Managing Director, In Corporate Pty Ltd (Chapter 13)

Dale Gietzelt, BA (Hons) PhD Grad Dip (Commerce, InfoMngt)
Senior Researcher, Health and Ageing Research Unit, South Eastern Sydney Area Health Service (Chapter 2)

Jill Gordon, MBBS BA MPM PhD FRACGP FACPM
Associate Professor, Associate Dean, Educational Development, Department of Medical Education, University of Sydney (Chapter 3)

Marianne Hammerton, MA
Executive Director, Department of Ageing, Disability and Home Care, Associate Fellow, Australian College of Health Services Executives (ACHSE) (Chapter 13)

Peter Harris, MBBS FRACGP
General Practitioner
Director, Curriculum Unit, Senior Lecturer, School of Public Health and Community Medicine, Faculty of Medicine, University of New South Wales (Chapter 7)

Gwyn Jones, BEd TESOL MEd (Admin)
Learning Advisor, Learning Centre, University of New South Wales (Chapter 2)

Max Kamien, AM Cit WA MBBS MD FRCP FRACP FRACGP FACRRM DPM DCH
Physician and general practitioner
Professor and Head, Department of General Practice, University of Western Australia (Chapter 11)

Alix Magney, BA (Sociology)
PhD candidate in School of Sociology, University of New South Wales, Sydney (Chapter 14)

Elizabeth O'Brien, Cert Nursing BNursing MPH
Senior Policy Officer, Australian Health Workforce Advisory Committee (Chapter 10)

Natalie O'Dea, BEc (Soc Sci) MEd
Consultant in health training (Chapters 1, 9, and 16)

Dimity Pond, BA Dip Ed MBBS Dip Soc Sci PhD FRACGP
Associate Professor, Head, Discipline of General Practice, University of Newcastle (Chapter 4)

Paul Sadler, BA (Hons) MSW
Chief Executive Officer, Aged and Community Services Association of New South Wales and Australian Capital Territory (Chapter 13)

Deborah Saltman, MBBS MD FRACGP FAFPHM
Professor, Head, General Practice Professorial Unit, Manly Hospital, University of Sydney (joint editor; author of Chapters 1, 9, and 16)

Kay Tucker, B Soc Sci (Lib)
Information Services Librarian, Law Library, Monash University (Chapter 5)

Martin B. Van Der Weyden, MD FRACP FRCPA
Editor, *The Medical Journal of Australia* (Chapter 12)

Patricia Youngblood, MA BA MEd PhD
Senior Lecturer, School of Public Health and Community Medicine, and Curriculum Unit, Faculty of Medicine, University of New South Wales (Chapter 6)

Preface

Communication skills are essential in health care. All practitioners listen to patients, interpret what they see and hear, remember what they have read and heard from others, and make sense of the information as they implement some type of health care process. This concise text follows the key information steps in health care. It covers both written and spoken communication, which are common elements in treatment contexts. Health care professionals from all disciplines should find *Communication for Health Care* useful. The text places communication in context, where professionals meet and work with patients, alongside other members of their own profession, and with members of different professions in one health care team.

Communication is more than conversations between two people. This text takes a broader definition of communication, and provides practical help for health care professionals, as they gather information, analyse it, and convey their conclusions and interpretations to others in ongoing professional contexts. Numerous small group and individual exercises are included, so that readers can further develop their communication skills, or simply revisit them as they fine-tune their health care practice.

This is an edited text, with contributions from experienced practitioners from different fields of health care, and from educators of the next generation of health care professionals. The chapters contain different views, rather than one dogma. Some chapters contain examples of theories and models. It is not intended that these be prescriptive. Rather, it is intended that readers be exposed to those views, and appreciate the diversity of perspectives. The contributors share a common concern: that communication is important for health care.

Communication for Health Care begins with the communicator; and the reader's own preference and style of communication with others is explored. The book canvasses cultural context and meaning of language and communication. In health care contexts, the process of meeting a patient is a central communication concern. This is introduced early in the book; the skills of listening and questioning are the focus. The next two chapters demonstrate that the interaction between carer and patient can be enhanced by the practitioner (and patient) being able to access diverse resources and information sources. For instance, the experience and wisdom of others is often contained in writings, which can be accessed by increasingly sophisticated communication tools. A collection of chapters follows on the analysis and communication process in a consultation, the partnership of carer and patient in reaching decisions, and the styles of interaction that may be chosen in health care relationships. The keeping of records on patient care, the verbal and written handing over of care, and the referral process from one institution to another are also explained. These systemic skills in communication are essential to effective management in health care. Communication processes between peers and within professional work teams are canvassed. The final few chapters focus on the skills of communicating with the media, preparing written resources for fellow professionals, and in publishing in professional forums. This is to communicate with the public and provide an ongoing resource for use in future communication episodes.

1

Starting with yourself

Catherine Berglund, Natalie O'Dea, and Deborah Saltman

We all need to recognise our own preferred way of communicating, and to recognise our strengths and weaknesses. We need to examine ourselves before we can become effective communicators with others. Different types of relationships can determine the appropriate mode of **communication**. Some choices of communication can already be made for us in different contexts. This chapter looks at us as social beings, and our capacities as effective social members, and team members.

Communication is a complex phenomenon. First, try to think of the complexity of communication in your own everyday life.

For instance, what characterises your home life? At home, do you live with others, or close by others, and communicate with them? Do you gather information on community activities, or distribute information? Are you busy with school events, and coordinating the busy schedules of others?

Think about the types of communication in which you are involved in your everyday life. Make a list of what you try to communicate to others, what others try to communicate to you, and how you do that. Do you speak face to face? Do you write letters or notes? Do you use communication devices like telephones or answering machines, or mechanisms like email? Do you enhance your reception of written communication by wearing glasses, or of aural communication by using a hearing aid?

As you think about the types of communication which you use, also think about the context of that communication. You may choose certain ways of communicating depending on the content of communication and appropriate options available to you. Sad news about friends for instance, is rarely communicated just on paper—it is far more common to speak to each other.

What do others think of you as a communicator? Do they thank you for listening? Do they think of you as rushed—and suggest catching up when you are not so busy? Do they find your notes hard to read or ambiguous? Do people tend to mix up where you plan to meet? Do you enjoy communicating with some people more than others? Is it because of successful past communication, or perhaps their encouraging manner?

Sometimes, systems of communication are set up that are intended to enhance communication. For instance, you have a post-box in your neighbourhood for posting letters to others. You have a mailbox at your house for receipt of mail from others. An organised system of collecting and delivering mail is an expected part of our communication options. An organised system of telephone lines is also expected. If these systems are disrupted, then communication options are disrupted. The systems are as much a communication concern as the individual interactions.

The style and manner of your interaction with others is of concern because it can affect the communication that is likely to result.

YOUR OWN COMMUNICATION STYLE

Recognising that we may have different behavioural styles and therefore varying needs in an interaction is a good starting point for more effective communication.

When we look at our own behavioural styles we can try to:

- understand how we communicate with others and recognise our own needs in an interaction
- recognise how our behaviour may be perceived by others and how it may affect them
- identify other people's preferred behavioural styles and needs, and subsequently modify our approach in order to communicate more effectively.

Behaviour is the 'tip of the iceberg'. It is what we see of other people. Under the surface lies much more; genetic traits, personality, life experiences, and attitudes. These aspects are less dynamic than behaviour. Behaviour is changeable according to the situation. For example, we would behave quite differently at a sporting event compared with how we would behave at home, or when sitting an examination, or at work.

Understanding a patient's behavioural style in any given consultation or preferred behavioural styles over a series of consultations helps us plan effective communications. Our own behavioural style as clinicians also affects our communication. Behavioural styles vary with the situations in which we find ourselves. In times of stress, we usually revert to our preferred style. Each style has its own unique features that may be viewed by the people we are communicating with in different ways, depending on what behavioural style they prefer.

We are going to describe a simple behavioural style model, but first it will be useful to ascertain what our preferred behavioural styles are in a specific situation. Two of us (Deborah Saltman and Natalie O'Dea) have done some work with a tool to use as you think about your behaviour style.[1] There are many other tools and models of behaviour. This is just one example.

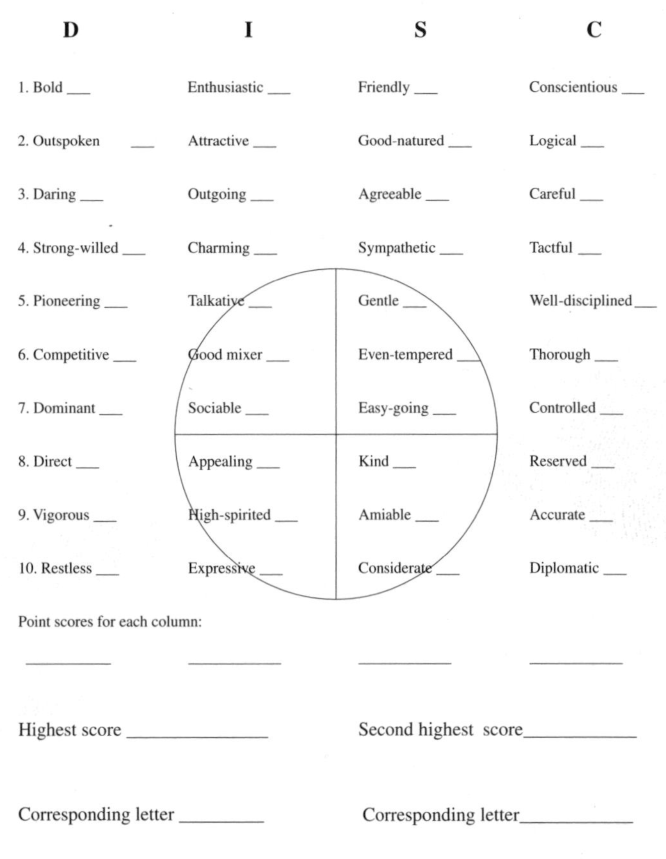

D	I	S	C
1. Bold ___	Enthusiastic ___	Friendly ___	Conscientious ___
2. Outspoken ___	Attractive ___	Good-natured ___	Logical ___
3. Daring ___	Outgoing ___	Agreeable ___	Careful ___
4. Strong-willed ___	Charming ___	Sympathetic ___	Tactful ___
5. Pioneering ___	Talkative ___	Gentle ___	Well-disciplined ___
6. Competitive ___	Good mixer ___	Even-tempered ___	Thorough ___
7. Dominant ___	Sociable ___	Easy-going ___	Controlled ___
8. Direct ___	Appealing ___	Kind ___	Reserved ___
9. Vigorous ___	High-spirited ___	Amiable ___	Accurate ___
10. Restless ___	Expressive ___	Considerate ___	Diplomatic ___

Point scores for each column:

___ ___ ___ ___

Highest score ___ Second highest score ___

Corresponding letter ___ Corresponding letter ___

To score the questionnaire, add up the total number of points in each of the four columns and write the point score in the space provided.

Figure 1.1 Questionnaire

Use the questionnaire in Figure 1.1 to identify your preferred behavioural style at work. The questionnaire contains ten lines, each comprised of four adjectives. In each line, rank the adjectives as to how accurately they describe how you behave in a work setting. Assign:

- 4 points to the word that best describes you
- 3 points to the word that is like you
- 2 points to the word that is a bit like you
- 1 point to the word that least describes you.

Do not spend a long time thinking about your answers, go with your first response. You may think that all of the adjectives describe you best, or that none of them do. This is a 'forced choice' questionnaire, so assign a point score to each adjective. When you have completed the questionnaire, each line should have a 1, 2, 3, and 4 point score in it. For example in the line:

1. Bold___ Enthusiastic___ Friendly___ Conscientious ___

if you think the adjective 'enthusiastic' describes you best, and 'bold' describes you least, with 'conscientious' a bit like you, and 'friendly' like you, your response would be as follows:

1. Bold *1* Enthusiastic *4* Friendly *3* Conscientious *2*

To score the questionnaire, add up the total number of points in each of the four columns and write the point score in the space provided. At the top of each column, there is a letter; D, I, S, or C. Write the letter at the top of the column that corresponds with your highest score in the space provided. Write the letter at the top of the column that corresponds with your second highest score in the space provided. These two letters correspond with your two preferred behavioural styles. You have a stronger preference for the style with the highest score, and a secondary preference for the style with the second highest score.

BEHAVIOURAL STYLE MODEL

The behavioural style model was originally developed by William Moulton Marston in the 1920s. He wrote about behaviour of people in his book entitled *Emotions of Normal People*.[2] Unlike his contemporaries Freud and Jung, Marston was interested in 'normal' people and their behaviour, as opposed to people with mental illness.

Many behavioural style models have arisen from Marston's work. Most of them describe behaviour in four distinct styles. The iteration we have used is called the DISC model. DISC is an acronym for the four behavioural styles: Direct, Influencing, Steady, and Conscientious.

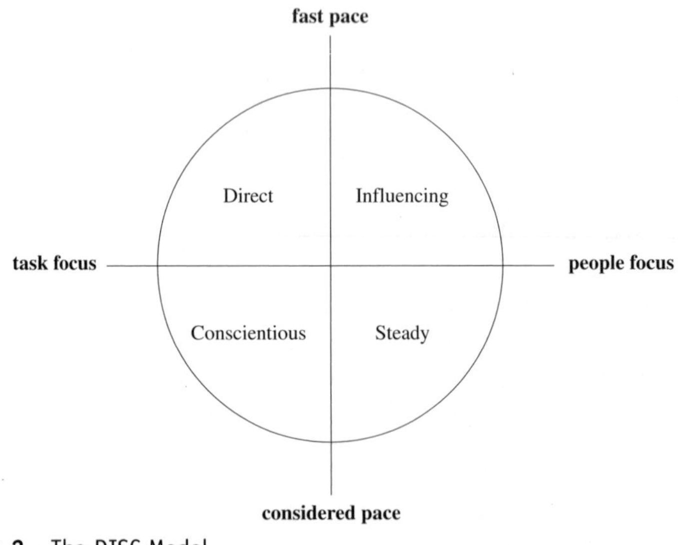

Figure 1.2 The DISC Model

The four styles are an interplay of our preferred focus (task or relationship focus) and the preferred pace at which we operate (fast or considered pace). The four behavioural styles are outlined as follows:

Direct

Characteristics of a person displaying a Direct behavioural style in a given situation are:

- focuses on tasks
- operates at a fast pace
- asks 'what?'
- likes making decisions
- is motivated to solve problems
- does not shirk confrontations
- accepts tasks as a personal challenge
- prefers direct answers
- questions the status quo
- acts independently.

May appear:

- insensitive
- unapproachable
- impatient.

Could do more of:

- listening
- considering and encouraging others
- developing greater patience.

When communicating with a person displaying a Direct behavioural style we should remember that this person needs us to:

- be brief and to the point
- be clear about expectations
- recognise their need for autonomy
- stick to the topic and eliminate time-wasters.

Influencing

Characteristics of a person displaying an Influencing behavioural style in a given situation are:

- focuses on people
- operates at a fast pace
- asks 'who?'
- is motivated to influence others
- expresses thoughts and feelings
- has infectious enthusiasm
- prefers working with people

- gives feedback easily
- is available for others.

May appear:

- superficial
- disorganised
- to lose interest.

Could do more of:

- attending to detail
- following through
- improving organisational skills.

When communicating with a person displaying an Influencing behavioural style we should remember that this person needs us to:

- be informal and sociable
- allow them to verbalise their thoughts and feelings
- use humour
- provide them with written details, try to keep them focused.

Steady

Characteristics of a person displaying a Steady behavioural style in a given situation are:

- focuses on people
- operates at a considered pace
- asks 'how?'
- is motivated to maintain harmony
- prefers participating in a group
- is a good team player
- listens more than talks
- is patient
- is easy to get along with.

May appear:

- resistant to change
- indecisive
- too open to the needs and opinions of others.

Could do more of:

- coping with change
- making decisions
- removing everyone else's problems from their shoulders.

When communicating with a person displaying a Steady behavioural style we should remember that this person needs us to:

- be systematic in our approach
- provide a consistent and secure environment
- explain thoroughly how things will be done
- let them adjust to change slowly.

Conscientious

Characteristics of a person displaying a Conscientious behavioural style in a given situation are:

- focuses on tasks
- operates at a considered pace
- asks 'why?'
- is motivated to achieve thoroughness
- prefers focusing on detail
- enjoys analysing things
- likes clearly defined goals
- is certain to follow standards closely
- aims for accuracy.

May appear:

- distant
- too fixed in their ways
- overly concerned with achieving perfection.

Could do more of:

- being open and more communicative
- learning how to deal with conflict
- accepting differences.

When communicating with a person displaying a Conscientious behavioural style we should remember that this person needs us to:

- give clear information and outline standards
- be precise and focused
- cut down on the socialising aspects
- show dependability and trustworthiness.

There is no best style of behaviour. We all have the capabilities to move between styles. Depending on the environment, the demands of a situation and the style of the person we are communicating with, we can modify our behaviour accordingly. We do, however, have a preferred style of behaviour and when placed under a stressful situation, we are more likely to revert to this more comfortable style.

BEHAVIOURAL STYLES IN CLINICAL PRACTICE

In a health care context, recognising our preferred behavioural styles and those of our patients can help us to conduct more effective clinical interactions. We can recognise how patients may perceive aspects of our behaviour, but more importantly by identifying a patient's behavioural style, we can recognise how best to transmit information and work towards what patients may want to achieve in a consultation.

Remember that:

- Direct-style patients like clinicians to be straightforward and open to their need for quick results.
- Influencing-style patients like clinicians to be friendly, emotionally honest, and to recognise their achievements.
- Steady-style patients like clinicians to be relaxed, agreeable, and cooperative.
- Conscientious-style patients like clinicians to be detailed and accurate.

Below are some points on how to identify and communicate with patients displaying the various behavioural styles in practice:

When a patient displaying Direct (task focus, fast pace) behaviour enters a consultation they may: be agitated about having had to wait in the waiting room to see the clinician; have a list of problems clearly identified they want to discuss; want the clinician to 'get straight to the point' and tell them what needs to be done to fix their health concern. If the clinician talks about relationship issues or tries to gain consensus rather than direct answers, this may be perceived as ineffectual and stalling behaviour. What this patient requires is a quick assessment, a concise knowledge update and a series of short, sharp strategies to deal with their concern. They want to get better quickly.

When a patient displaying Influencing (people focus, fast pace) behaviour enters a consultation they may: have already spoken to everyone in the waiting room; want to talk with the clinician about their social calendar rather than their presenting health concern; have difficulty focusing on one particular problem. If the clinician cuts them off in the middle of their socialising or expression of their feelings, this may be perceived as uncaring and 'clinical'. This patient requires a quick response to the social aspects raised and health concerns. The patient may need to be focused on the relevant issues. They may also require instructions for follow-through.

When a patient displaying Steady (people focus, considered pace) behaviour enters a consultation they may: not mind having had to wait to see the clinician (they may have offered their appointment time for other patients in a hurry); want to know how their health concern may affect other people, for example, whether it is contagious; ask how established a particular treatment is within the medical profession; and if the medication is new they may ask how many other patients have used it. If the clinician is too direct and hurried in their approach, this may be perceived by this patient as bossy and unfeeling. This patient requires a series of community- , family- , or group-based strategies to deal with their problem. This patient also needs time to adjust to changes in their health care.

When a patient displaying Conscientious (task focus, considered pace) behaviour enters a consultation they may: know precisely how long they have been waiting to see the clinician; have a comprehensive list of issues they want to discuss in detail; bring information about therapies or information from the Internet they want answers to. If the clinician does not answer this patient's questions in sufficient detail, they may find the interaction scatty and incomplete. What this patient requires are all the details about their health problem and its management. They would like to know the follow-up procedures and time-frames involved. This patient requires structure and a methodical approach to their condition.

TRAINING ISSUES

Given that communication is a factor in being an effective health care professional, and that it is not as straightforward a skill as it seems, it is not surprising that development of communication skills is addressed in training. Professionals in training can expect to be assessed on their communication ability, and to receive some opportunities for developing effective communication strategies. The way communication is achieved is as much a concern as the content of communication.

The process of communication is a developmental issue. Professionals need to have developed a sense of self and be able to empathise with others for instance. They need to be able to cope with large amounts of information, which is sometimes incomplete or apparently conflicting. This is why, traditionally, communication ability is viewed as intertwined with identity formation and cognitive capacity. Regardless of which developmental model you agree with, it is clear that there is a process of learning to handle increasingly difficult communication tasks.

The following is one view of the complexity in clinical communication:

- taking a history, and using basic questioning techniques
- interviewing, using more open-ended styles
- giving information to patients
- accepting responsibility for a patient
- developing a close relationship with a patient
- collaborating or negotiating with a patient
- handling difficult interviews, and difficult material in interviews
- relating effectively with 'difficult' people
- becoming a healer.[3]

You will have noticed that these focus on personal interaction in interview settings. That has traditionally been the focus for developing communication skills. Notice also, however, that even in this list, professional access to resources and appropriate synthesis of material is crucial to the giving of information to the patient. You will also sense the importance of communication as a way of dealing with a patient over time.

Interview and interaction skills

Interview and personal interaction skills are vital for health care professionals, who work with individual clients on personal health concerns. The success of a clinical relationship is dependent on clear and open communication of the health concerns, and of options for assessment and management. Interpersonal processes and interviewing skills are commonly thought of as the two main components of communicative behaviours.

Interpersonal processes usually focus on the nature of interpersonal interaction between one professional and one client. This can be managed by the professional, to some extent, by setting the tone of the interaction. Use of different language and speech patterns can affect the social nature of a relationship.[4] Establishing 'rapport' sets up an interpersonal process of trust.

Interviewing skills related to content are about the gathering, synthesis, and provision of information during a clinical interview. This is more than receiving information from a client. It is facilitating that information, and also facilitating exchange of information, from professional to client. Interviewing skills related to technique are about the competence of the interviewer. At a minimum, the interviewer needs to be proficient in managing the interview, including effective opening and closing of the interview, choice of open-ended and closed questions, listening skills, and behaviours that establish rapport.[5] Two chapters in particular are devoted to this facility to manage an interview: Chapter 3 by Jill Gordon and Chapter 4 by Dimity Pond.

So, at a minimum, the basic communication skills needed for clinical interviewing are:

- how to begin and end an interview
- active listening
- facilitation by appropriate use of questions
- identifying and responding to verbal and non-verbal cues.

Some training programs concentrate on these basic skills, and students practise them in role-play, rehearse them by watching others and video demonstrations, and providing feedback. The practice can be on difficult communication, such as breaking bad news and dealing with anger from patients, as well as more routine consultations. These training programs are thought to be successful, with even brief training improving communication ability. The challenge for trainers then is to reinforce skills throughout training. A caution is that personal confidence is no guarantee of competence.[6] Students recognise that actual practice is a must.[7] You should be prepared to practise, rather than just read through this text. Some exercises are provided to facilitate that process for you.

Small group work is frequently used to develop communication skills and interview techniques. Students are encouraged to observe effective role models, and this observation is extended into role-play. Davies and Farmer have described the communication-skills group leader in a small group as holding three roles: guardian, in encouraging participation in a safe environment; resource person, to share their knowledge and experience with the group; and role model of appropriate behaviour.[8]

This can be gradually developed in hypothetical situations in which the student acts as the professional, with simulated patients. The use of simulated patients provides an opportunity for rehearsal of communication skills with real people pretending to be patients. This gives students the freedom to try things out, and even make mistakes, as they develop their own effective communication capability. In programs that use simulated patients, a gradual improvement in skill is reported.[9]

Simulated patients are commonly used to assess a trainee's level of communication skill. In a communication-skills program in Switzerland for internal medicine residents, patient-centred communication skills such as active listening and inviting patient participation in decision-making were assessed before and after by way of videotaped interviews with simulated patients. Improvement for those in the training course was observed.[10]

The study of particular communication skills is well established in nursing practice. In discussions with patients, being able to facilitate patient disclosure of key concerns was found to depend on the nurse's use of open directive questions, questions with psychological focus, and clarification of psychological aspects, rather than specific closed physiologically focused questions.[11]

As well as practical experience, students also need to understand, on a theoretical level, the options and rationales for types of communication exchanges and communication choices in consultations, and have a positive attitude to using your repertoire of skills.[12]

When an interaction develops into a series of consultations, the management of that interaction over time is crucial. Deborah Saltman and Natalie O'Dea suggest a way of managing interaction in Chapter 9. The partnership of interaction and information exchange is also a feature of Chapter 8 by Catherine Berglund.

These concepts of individual interpersonal interaction and interview skills can be extended to teams of professionals. An atmosphere of trust in a clinical unit is obviously enhanced by a pattern of good rapport with individual team members. The effective sharing of information between team members is an issue of handover and note-keeping, and referral. This is dealt with in Chapter 10 by Elizabeth O'Brien and in Chapter 11 by Max Kamien.

COMMUNICATION ON THE JOB

Communication is an increasing focus in the modern health care curricula, and the approach is far beyond teaching basic interviewing skills. There is now a tendency to look at the broad sense of what is required of the professional on the job, defining learning outcomes which are needed for 'competent and reflective' practitioners, and then including those facets in training programs. Communication is a feature of the health care professional's work.

Basic communication skills have been listed by a group of medical educators to include dealing with:

- patients
- relatives
- colleagues
- agencies
- media/press

as well as:

- teaching
- managing
- patient advocacy
- mediation and negotiation

by telephone or in writing.[13]

In a competency-based model of education, the importance of what the professional is able to do, technically, is central, but how professionals approach their practice, and the personal attributes of the person performing the work, are the defining aspects of the professional. So, these communication abilities would permeate other technical tasks, such as those of history taking, in clinical skills, patient management, and information handling skills in patient records and professional resources. The appropriate and sensitive application of all of these skills defines the professional in practice.

On the flip side, poor communication skills can inhibit the performance of other technical skills. For instance, diagnostic efficiency is doubtful if there is a failure to elicit full, relevant information from a patient.[14]

This text adopts the broader view of communication. Apart from chapters on medical records, and handover and referral, noted above, chapters on the media, and organisational issues and team work, are included as Chapter 15 by Peter Baume and Alix Magney, and Chapter 13 by Marianne Hammerton, Paul Sadler, and Alan Cartwright. Written communication for patients and fellow professionals is covered in Chapters 15 by Catherine Berglund, and Chapter 16 by Natalie O'Dea and Deborah Saltman. The gathering of information is the subject of Chapter 5 by Kay Tucker.

While there is training for the professional to be ready for the communication in health contexts, there is often little preparation for the individual patient. Each person presents with their own facility in communication, language, and capacity for complex thought. Being aware of language and cultural concerns is essential, as discussed in Dale Gietzelt and Gwyn Jones' chapter, 'What language?'. Health care professionals must also be prepared to deal with many variations in personality and communication styles. In a way, professionals need to have a repertoire of management and responses at the ready.

As a way of reviewing this chapter, try the following exercise.

Communication Challenge Exercise

Using the following questions as a guide, identify a challenge in your workplace:

1 What have you achieved?
2 What communication strategies have helped you achieve this?
3 What more do you want to achieve?
4 How does your communication need to modify to help you achieve these aims?
5 How does your behavioural style need to modify according to the situation?

NOTES

1 *DiSC Dimensions of Behaviour.* Carlson Learning Company, Minneapolis, Min., 1996.

2 Marston, W.M. *Emotions of Normal People.* Ormskirk, Lancs, Lyster, 1989 (first published 1928).

3 Weston, W.W. and Lipkin, M. Doctors learning communication skills: developmental issues, in M. Stewart and B. Roter (eds) *Communicating with Medical Patients.* Newbury Park, Cal., Sage Publishers, 1989, pp. 43–57.

4 Anderson, L.A. and Sharpe, P.A. Improving patient and provider communication: A synthesis and review of communication intervention, *Patient Education and Counseling,* 1991, vol. 17, pp. 99–134, p. 102.

5 Anderson, L.A. and Sharpe, P.A. Improving patient and provider communication: A synthesis and review of communication intervention, *Patient Education and Counseling,* 1991, vol. 17, pp. 99–134, p. 102.

6 Marteau, T.M., Humphrey, C., Matoon, G., Kidd, J., Lloyd, M. and Horder, J. Factors influencing the communication skills of first-year clinical medical students, *Medical Education,* 1991, vol. 25, pp. 127–34, p. 129.

7 Usherwood, T. Subjective and behavioural evaluation of the teaching of patient interview skills, *Medical Education,* 1993, vol. 27, pp. 41–7, p. 43.

8 Davies, P.G. and Farmer, E.A. Teaching communication skills in small groups, *Medical Journal of Australia,* 1992, vol. 156, pp. 259–60.

9 Duerson, M.C., Romrell, L.J. and Stevens, C.B. Impacting faculty teaching and student performance: nine years' experience with the Objective Structured Clinical Examination, *Teaching & Learning in Medicine,* 2000, vol. 12, no. 4 pp. 176–82.

10 Langewitz, W.A., Eich, P., Kiss, A. and Wossmer, B. Improving communication skills—a randomized controlled behaviorally oriented intervention study for residents in internal medicine, *Psychosomatic Medicine,* 1988, vol. 60, no. 3 pp. 268–73.

11 Booth, K., Maguire, P. and Hillier, V. F. Measurement of communication skills in cancer care: myth or reality? *Journal of Advanced Nursing,* 1999, vol. 30, no. 5 pp. 1073–9.

12 Evans, B.J., Sweet, B. and Coman, G.J. Behavioural assessment of the effectiveness of a communication programme for medical students, *Medical Education,* 1993, vol. 27, pp. 344–50.

13 Harden, R.M., Crosby, J.R., Davis, M.H. and Friedman, M. AMEE Guide No. 14: Outcome-based education: Part 5—From competency to meta-competency: a model for the specification of learning outcomes, *Medical Teacher,* 1999, vol. 21, no. 6, pp. 546–52, p. 548.

14 Evans, B.J., Stanley, R.O., Mestrovic, R. and Rose L. Effects of communication skills training on students' diagnostic efficiency, *Medical Education,* 1991, vol. 25, pp. 517–26.

2

What language?

Dale Gietzelt and Gwyn Jones

The choice of language for communication presents as a stumbling block for many people. We come from all over the world to train and work together. Finding common ground and ensuring that we are skilled and fluent in the chosen language are essential in health care. Key areas to be checked to guard against miscommunication are outlined. Health care workers all know how challenging and rewarding it can be to work with patients from other **cultures** and with other languages. Sometimes, the language hurdle faced in this situation by the health care professional needs expert assistance. Interpreter use is examined, and practical steps are given for interpreting with patients in health care treatment situations.

WHAT IS LANGUAGE?

It was once believed that if you knew the vocabulary of a language you could communicate in that language.[1] We now know this is not accurate. This misconception still prevails and results in many speakers of a second language finding understanding and meaning difficult when initially immersed in a second-language culture. This same frustration is often mirrored by members of the first-language culture who find themselves repeating the same words, increasing the volume with each utterance and expecting these strategies to result in successful communication. This is often simplistically evaluated as a language problem. But what do we mean by the term 'language'?

Simply, language can be seen as a system of shared symbols governed by sets of rules. Language is made up of two intricately woven parts: verbal and non-verbal cues. Neither functions without the other. They work as a team to produce meaning. Verbal communication takes the form of the written and spoken word while non-verbal communication conveys meaning without the use of words.

In the health care setting, the health care user–practitioner relationship is

> built through communication and the effective use of language. Along with clinical reasoning, observations, and non-verbal cues, skilful use of language endows the history with its clinical power and establishes the clinical tool as the clinician's most powerful tool ... Language is the means by which a [practitioner] accesses a patient's beliefs about health and illness ... creating an opportunity to address and reconcile different belief systems. Furthermore, it is through language that [practitioners] and patients achieve an empathetic connection that may be therapeutic in itself.[2]

The realisation of effective communication through language is not as straightforward as it is presented here. In a study involving 500 patients of 74 American physicians, the component of the medical encounter deemed second most important to patients, and sixth to physicians, was the communication of medical information.[3] Indeed, *'health professionals frequently underestimate patients' desire for and ability to cope with information'*.[4] Thus the practitioner needs to learn how to *impart* information to users as much as *elicit* information from them. This is true with communication *between* practitioners as much as in the user–practitioner encounter. Language expressed between professionals will clearly diverge from that between user and professional; not only will the level of esoteric knowledge and jargon vary, but the power relations between participants will also differ. Nowhere is this more apparent than when participants of an encounter do not share a common language and/or cultural foundation. Furthermore, while language and culture are intermeshed as social practice, individuals within a cultural subgroup can manifest uniqueness and heterogeneity.[5] Thus, language serves as *'a vessel of individual and collective social experience'*.[6]

This chapter will explore the complexity of language as a communication tool in the health care context. Activities are provided that will help build a personal awareness of you as a health practitioner, in your personal communication style. Spoken language, written language, non-verbal language, sign language, and the role of the interpreter are examined.

The questions in Box 2.1 are designed to allow you to reflect on how we individually take ownership of our personal, social, and professional language, with our own culture and style of communication.

Language as communication

We see communication as a process of negotiation, of the participants' jostling to find the right fit between them. The challenge often arises when the symbols of the shared language seem to be the same but the values and beliefs are different. A perceived fit may actually produce a misfit resulting in a miscommunication. There is potential for miscommunication within any relationship, whether personal or professional, or between a first-language culture and second-

Box 2.1: Activity 1

Exploring these concepts requires an awareness and reflection of personal perceptions of what language means to you. It is this awareness that may help lead to a common understanding. Use the following focus questions to help you think about language.

- How would you define language?
- How do you feel about language?
- How does language work for you?
- How has language worked against you?
- How do you decide which language to use?

language culture. In fact, miscommunication is part of the overall communication process. The use of language and the awareness of culture are an integral part of this process being successful, since fruitful communication results in shared meaning and understanding. However, confirmation of the vital stage of understanding is often overlooked. The classic question 'Do you understand?' is often responded to in the affirmative; however, the opposite may actually be the case. A simple strategy to overcome this is to compose a question that allows your communication partner to actively reconstruct and describe their understanding of the situation in their own words. Questions such as 'Tell me ...?' or 'What are you going to ...?' or 'What do you know about ...?' allow both partners to check the shared concepts and understandings of a specific situation.

Between colleagues, common communication pitfalls include defining roles and boundaries, and disparate philosophies of care.[7] External constraints also have a role to play in whether the flow of information between people remains free and open in the context of the medical or health encounter. There is

Box 2.2: Activity 2

Think of a time when you were aware of a miscommunication occurring. Describe the situation in as much detail as possible.

- What topic was being discussed?
- Where did it take place?
- Who was involved?
- What time of day was it?
- Why do you think the miscommunication took place?
- What part did language and culture play in this situation?

evidence of clinical errors occurring often, due to ineffective communication between health care team members.[8] In addition, with consultation times limited, there is often insufficient time to fully explain the condition, treatment options, and expected outcomes. One way around this is to ensure users have access to written or audiovisual resources for gleaning further information.[9] This of course presupposes many points: literacy; competence in a language in which the material is available; use of plain language, not jargon; access to and competency in the use of the technology to see or hear the audiovisual resource; and capacity to comprehend complex processes and ideas.

But it is not only external constraints that affect the flow of communication. According to Maher,[10] physicians seldom give users more than about ten to fifteen seconds to respond to a question. When communication flow falters because of language difficulties and poor compliance, inappropriate follow-up and patient dissatisfaction often result.[11] Research shows that there is a direct correlation between effective communication and improved health outcomes.[12]

Language and culture

The partnership of language and culture is the active process of relationship building that results in successful and sustained communication among health professionals and health care users.[13] As in any relationship, an awareness of interpersonal skills and the recognition of possible differences between the players enhance this social process. It is the responsibility of all those involved to negotiate a common meaning and understanding. This awareness is of increasing importance as the global community expands and we live and work within a broader cultural community.

So how does this partnership of language and culture work? How do we come to this shared meaning? As stated earlier, we perceive language as a system of shared symbols regulated by certain rules. Culture is a complex set of values, beliefs, norms, customs, rules, and codes that socially define people and give them a sense of commonality.[14] On one hand, we have the tools of our language, that is, words, and on the other, our perceptions and definitions of what is taking place, imbued with the knowledge gained from our own experiences. This union is what produces meaning.

Thus, if working in a community comprising culturally and/or linguistically non-mainstream people, it is useful for health professionals to learn not only about the prevailing cultural practices and language(s) in the area, but also the differing beliefs about health and illness. Understanding a patient's culturally determined disease model might be essential to the provision of quality care.[15]

It is important to recognise that biomedicine, too, is a culturally constructed (Western) phenomenon, emerging as it did from Cartesian notions of the separation of mind and body. Biomedicine is rooted in capitalism, which highlights individualism and commodification of relations and services, continuing this tradition with:

- biological reductionism, in which disease is traced back to the smallest possible elements (such as DNA or genes), all located within the individual; and
- expensive but indispensable pharmaceuticals and technology.

Issues of power come into play since biomedicine is premised on the ethnocentric assumption that science is the only appropriate basis and authority for practice. Other forms of health care, whether traditional or alternative, are often relegated to the domain of mere 'beliefs', not absolute 'truths' or 'facts'.

People from non-Western cultures traditionally hold different beliefs about the cause, nature, and necessary treatment of illness. Medico-religious traditions of Southeast Asia, for example, attribute illness to possession by spirits.[16] Wilson and Billones,[17] focusing on Filipino culture, explain the basis of a belief system related to religious practice, wherein followers practise an acceptance of life events as being beyond an individual's control. One should accept unquestioningly what life brings, as personal destiny or God's will. This reflects strongly an external locus of control. A related value concerns interpersonal communication. Maintaining harmony and avoiding confrontation are particularly desirable. O'Hara and Zhan believe an understanding of cultural/philosophical frameworks such as Confucianism elucidates why elderly people from Chinese backgrounds are opposed to eradicative surgery (according to the need to return the body in its wholeness, to ensure a proper afterlife).[18] It also explains why Buddhist people refuse heavy narcotics in palliative care (in order to steer consciously and actively the precarious route through death to the best destination that their karma allows).

Some of the other causes to which illness is attributed are as follows:

- the condition of the blood: among certain African Americans and in Chinese and Ayurvedic medicine;[19]
- imbalances of 'hot' and 'cold' forces in the body: with the Chinese, Mexicans, Puerto Ricans, and Haitians;
- social indiscretions or deviances (such as offending another person or not fulfilling social obligations): many traditional African peoples;[20]
- a fright (*susto*): many Latin American societies;[21] or,
- transgressions from past lives or possession by evil spirits: among the Vietnamese and other Southeast Asian peoples.[22]

Presentation and expression of symptoms may also be culturally determined. Middle Eastern and Mediterranean people may voice the pain quite emotionally, as it is believed refraining from one's pain only aggravates the illness, while indigenous Americans and Southeast Asians behave stoically.

Even the ways illness, disease and/or negative outcomes are addressed differ across cultures. Hudgings discusses how adverse medication effects, complications from procedures, advance directives and death are best communicated using the third person plural among the Navajo: 'when *people* do this, *they* might get that' replaces 'if *you* do this, *you* might get that.'[23]

In traditional Hispanic societies, all health care decisions are family decisions, but the degree to which this occurs may differ according to class and the rural/urban divide.[24] It makes sense, therefore, to take the time to find out about patients, both as individuals and as members of an ethnic group. It may take some time, but it is worth the effort required to learn about people's culturally specific ideas of health and illness if compliance and positive treatment outcomes are the goal.

Thus, communication can in reality commence before the actual encounter. In the following sections, the various communication vehicles—the spoken word, written communication, non-verbal communication, and sign language (from the limited experience of hearing people)—will be examined.

THE SPOKEN WORD

As mentioned previously, the language used in communication between health professionals differs from that used with health care users. Language between practitioners is often laced with jargon and assumed knowledge. But even here it cannot be assumed that the flow of communication is open. Benner, for example has demonstrated how a nurse expert's clinical, contextual, and intuitive judgement is sometimes incomprehensible to the novice who has been trained with rule-based practice and linear thinking.[25]

To patients/users, language is used to convey certain underlying messages. In order to defuse technical terms, many medical practitioners use the 'what they call' phrase, as in *'It looks to me just like what they call a cervical erosion… '*.[26] This effectively distances the physician from the scientist, through an alignment with the patient/user in an 'us-and-them' situation. The use of diminishing phrases such as 'just', 'only' and 'a little' reduces the threat of potentially more serious problems in the presenting complaint to the patient/user, as in *'it's only a little virus'* or *'you've had this pain just for a few days?'* A perceived threat is kept to a minimum and, according to Skelton and Hobbs, patients/users perceive that they do not need to worry. This language of diminution and emotion is what these authors call a 'therapeutic use of language'.

When delivering bad news, language and how the information is imparted are crucial. Delivery should be at the patient's own pace.[27] It should begin with a warning shot, such as *'I'm afraid I have bad news'*. Hope should always be conveyed, but within the context of truthfulness. While in Western cultures, patients and family members prefer to have complete information, this may not be the case with persons of other cultural backgrounds. Simple language without euphemisms or jargon that tend to confuse the listeners is suggested, along with some form of documentation of available resources, all delivered gradually.[28]

Language and how the information is imparted are also important for setting boundaries to the encounter. For instance, to signify the finishing of an event or consultation, an 'exit ceremony' needs to be in place,[29] one that is mutually recognisable as such.

All these issues reach another level of complexity when the patient does not speak English at all or only at a superficial level. This is particularly so when language competence is confused with intellectual ability.[30]

The activity in box 2.3 can be explored by taping an interaction. First, seek permission from all involved, record and try to be as natural as possible. Play back the tape and try to identify the various types of language you have used. Awareness of both the language you use and the situations in which you use it can help both to develop a sensitivity to your audience and to determine which language will be most effective.

Box 2.3: Activity 3

In thinking about spoken communication, try to answer the following questions:

- How do I speak to people in my professional, social, and personal contexts?
- What is different?
- How does my language change?
- What language do I use? (Refer to the verbal stocktake in Table 2.1.)

Table 2.1: Verbal stocktake

Professional language	technical language, jargon, buzz words, abbreviations, acronyms
Social language	metaphors, colloquialisms, regional words, idiomatic phrases, similes, metaphors
Personal language	slang, euphemisms, clichés, proverbs

THE USE OF INTERPRETERS

Language can inhibit full participation in health services. It is recognised, for instance, as a key obstacle to non-English-speaking women's attendance at a British cervical screening program.[31] In another study, patient compliance rates were shown to rise considerably when an interpreter service was incorporated into a health centre encompassing a large migrant population in Canada.[32] It seems therefore that quality of patient care can be improved when steps are taken to enhance language facilities for patients from non-English-speaking backgrounds (NESB). The provision of, or common access to, interpreter services is thus an essential element of both effective health care and positive treatment outcomes.

In areas of high NESB populations, clinicians tend to rely on one of six mechanisms to communicate with patients:

1 Their own language skills

Using one's own language skills is of course the best alternative, provided the health care professional is fluent in the required language. One study of resident physicians who had undertaken a 45-hour medical Spanish program in the USA found that significant errors occurred even when these doctors believed their language proficiency was adequate.[33] Use of inadequate language skills may therefore compromise efficient information transfer and distract the clinician's intellectual focus away from clinical matters,[34] thereby affecting outcomes.

2 Language skills of a bilingual health worker

Bilingual health workers remove the need for calling in interpreters, and therefore save time and money. However, there is no guarantee that someone will be available when required.[35] It would be hoped that such health workers had received some minimal training in professional interpreting.

3 The skills of family or friends

The perceived advantages of using these people are their ready availability, the fact that they may have knowledge of the presenting problem, and that their presence may be reassuring to the patient/user. However, the risk is that such a person may not stop his or her own views from colouring the translation. They may try to protect the patient/user from bad news or withhold information about side effects, believing it may contribute to compliance. The patient may also wish to withhold embarrassing or stigmatising information.[36]

In particular, children fluent in English should not be used, for various reasons:

- some of the information to be relayed may be embarrassing for them;[37]
- some of the information to be relayed may contain biomedical words or concepts with which the child is not familiar;
- the professional may not glean the full picture of why the patient is presenting as there may be some information the child should not know (for example a woman may not say she has pain during sexual intercourse if her young son is interpreting for her); and,
- using children as interpreters distorts the family power and responsibility structure.[38]

Confidentiality may—or may be perceived to—be breached if a member of the local community is used for interpreting.

4 *Ad hoc* (untrained) interpreters

Although some of these (usually non-clinical staff or volunteers within a hospital or clinic setting) may have an instinctive understanding of what is required of them, others may exhibit ineptness owing to lack of empathy or insufficient grasp of the language.[39] Ebden, Carey, Bhatt, and Harrison found that between 23 and 52 per cent of words and phrases in their study were inaccurately translated by *ad hoc* interpreters, such as family members, friends, or hospital employees.[40]

5 Trained interpreters

If a clinician is not familiar with a particular language, or is uncomfortable with the potential for information distortion that can occur through an untrained interpreter, then only trained professionals should be used.[41] These interpreters maintain a strict code of confidentiality, and are trained in *'interpreting the sense and intent of what is said while preserving the content of the interview'*.[42]

It should be remembered that the cross-cultural or -linguistic health encounter represents a sharing of the control of the interview with the interpreter. This person is in a position of considerable power as a cultural agent and a two-way channel of information. As a professional, an interpreter is trained to be neutral, but neutrality cannot be guaranteed.[43] Using interpreters can be problematic due to class distinctions, ethnic rivalry, cultural differences, and other power differentials in the home country. Thus, while ideally an interpreter functions neutrally and does not influence decision-making, the clinician needs to stay attuned to possible tensions and hesitancies on the part of the participants.

6 Telephone interpreters

If a trained interpreter is not available on site, then a telephone interpreter should be sought. They are immediately accessible, saving time and resources. The disadvantage of telephone interpreting is that the interpreter cannot see a patient's non-verbal communication, and it is therefore much harder for both patient and health professional. One advantage, however, is that patient confidence in the consultation's confidentiality may be enhanced when an interpreter is not present, particularly if the interpreter is recruited from the patient's local ethnic community.[44] In other words, anonymity can be maintained.

When an interpreter is booked, the health care provider must state exactly what language the patient speaks—saying a patient is Indian, for example. is not useful. At the beginning of the interview, the interpreter should be introduced to the patient, their role explained, and confidentiality stressed.[45] The health care professional should not direct questions to the interpreter but to the patient.

Questions like *'Ask him when his pain commenced'* should therefore be avoided; rather, the question should be directed at the patient, as if the interpreter were not present: *'When did your pain commence?'* Seating should be in the form of a triangle. Attentiveness and eye contact should be maintained with the patient, with the interpreter seen more as a neutral tool to achieving an outcome than a participant in the encounter. As Phelan and Parkman point out, this contributes to the sense of direct communication.[46] When the interpreter is translating, an occasional nod or look of understanding helps to keep the lines of communication open, as does a response to a non-verbal cue. The clinician should pause frequently, reiterate and summarise important facts, and at times ask the patient to repeat what has been said for confirmation of comprehension. The patient should be encouraged to ask questions and say if something is unclear. Throughout the interview, the clinician needs to maintain control and direction, and recognise that the interpreter is only supposed to intervene to clarify or check meaning.

For physical examinations, the patient must consent to the presence of the interpreter. If the interpreter is not present, care needs to be taken beforehand to explain the procedures involved. After the patient has left, the clinician may care to discuss the meeting with the interpreter and check any queries that emerged, particularly when the meeting has been emotionally draining. Any such discussion should be about communication issues, not the patient, so as to maintain confidentiality and respect. Any further consultations with this patient should comprise the same interpreter, wherever possible.[47]

In psychiatric interviews, interpreters should be warned that the interview may take longer than normal, and that it might be emotionally distressing. If the patient is psychotic and likely to say things that might not make immediate sense, the interpreter should be informed.[48]

THE WRITTEN WORD

There are many advantages to written language.[49] Written language allows for the distribution and uniformity of directions and instruction and has the advan-

Box 2.4: Activity 4

Use this activity to explore your own written communication.

- Why do you write?
- When do you write?
- Who is your target readership/audience?
- How would you describe your own writing style?
- How easy is it to read your writing script?
- Do you enjoy writing?

tage of being able to be reread and thought through. It also provides a (permanent) record of communication.

Written material is frequently provided to patients. However, since recent literature highlights the fact that up to 62 per cent of certain clinical populations may be unable to read or understand medical instructions, **illiteracy** features as an obstacle to positive health outcomes.[50] Many persons with poor reading skills have developed various methods for concealing their illiteracy,[51] so health care professionals should not assume their patients can read. Apparent non-compliance may not be intended non-compliance. Such patients need explicit oral instructions as well as written material to take home. Audiovisual material may also be useful. If the patient does not speak English, it should not be assumed that they are at least literate in their own **language**, as this may not be the case.

To evaluate the clarity of your writing it is important to be aware of your specific audience and to write for a decided purpose. The use of the Fog Index is a simple strategy that assesses the readability of a written text.[52] The lower the Fog Index score, the easier the text is to understand and the wider the potential readership/audience. *Time* magazine has a Fog Index of 10, which approximates the reading level of a young adult. Postgraduate academic texts in specialised fields score around 18. Once the score is more than 20, the text is seen as incomprehensible.

As well as traditional forms of writing, electronic mail or email can be used as a vehicle of communication between health care professionals and patients,

Box 2.5: Activity 5

To evaluate your own writing, choose a paragraph aimed at a specific audience and follow the steps below.

To calculate the average length of the sentence in a section of text:

1 Note the number of words in each successive sentence and subtotal as you go.
2 Stop with the sentence that ends nearest the 100 word total.
3 Divide the total number of words in the passage by the number of sentences.

To calculate the percentage of difficult words in a passage:

1 Count the number of words of 3 syllables or more per 100 words.
2 Do not include proper nouns, compound words, verb forms where 'es' or 'ed' result in 3 syllable verbs.

To calculate the Fog Index of your writing:

1 Add the average length and the number of 3 syllable or more words and multiply by 0.4.
2 To reduce the Fog Index in your writing, aim to write shorter sentences, using fewer noun groups and increasing the frequency of verbs.

and between professionals themselves. It has the advantage of being able to pass the same piece of information to different people simultaneously.[53] Physicians appear to be approaching the Internet with a degree of caution. A 1997 survey of practitioners found that the Internet was primarily used for clinical research, followed by physician-to-physician communication, displaying judicious use in patient matters,[54] for fear of security breaches. Protection of the privacy of the data communicated is an important issue. Encryption software can assist in preventing interception.[55] Cost-effectiveness is reported to be a compelling reason for the use of email in the medical encounter.[56] Not only does it save patients' time and money, but also physicians may find certain patients to be better managed out of the office, freeing up available time to see other patients.

Email is a great leveller inasmuch as it carries little information about the social status, hierarchical position, race, age, or position of the sender. Language tends to be less formal and more conversational in style than conventional letters. For some email users, body language and tone of voice are conveyed by 'smileys' or 'emoticons', where :) or :-) signifies happy; :-D signifies laughing; :- (means sad; and ;-) indicates winking. Other shorthand includes FYI (for your information) and BTW (by the way).[57] ALL CAPITAL LETTERS IN AN EMAIL MESSAGE signifies shouting.[58]

NON-VERBAL LANGUAGE

Non-verbal language is simply defined as the communication of meaning without the use of the written or spoken word. This relationship between verbal and non-verbal, however, is not a balanced one. *'In a normal two person conversation, the verbal components carry less than 35% of the social meaning of the situation; more than 65% of the social meaning is carried on the non-verbal band.'*[59]

This imbalance demands an awareness that saying *'I told them'* does not mean effective communication has taken place. Since health care professionals cannot speak every language, they need to be aware that their body can speak eloquently for them. Non-verbal language, the process by which people communicate their emotions in non-verbal ways, conveys important messages that the speaker and listener exchange unconsciously. It encompasses paralinguistic cues, which include cries, laughter, sighs, groans, intonation and tone of voice, that are vocal, but not verbal sounds.[60] Looking people in the eyes when talking, facing them and keeping one's palms open and relaxed are all indications of sincerity, while the opposites, as well as pulling the ears and touching the mouth or nose, signify the exact truth is not being told. Assertions of power can be seen in such mannerisms as speaking imperatively, gesticulating near or pointing at a person (especially with a pen or instrument in one's hand) and standing haughtily.[61] For example, studies have shown that nurses' body language can convey to the patient that they are not interested in what is being said; this could occur when nurses are in a hurry or if they avoid being in close proximity to the patient.[62] Patients can feel depersonalised and excluded through nurses' tone of voice, use of short sentences, rushed movements, lack of eye contact or 'deadpan' facial expressions.[63] What is interesting about non-verbal language is that *all* humans use it to communicate, including people with speech impairments and babies. However, it is important to note that, while certain gestures are instinctive and universal, such as crying and smiling, others are culturally determined. Bulgarians and Greeks, for instance, may signal 'no' by nodding and 'yes' by shaking their heads from side to side, unlike most other peoples of the world.[64]

Non-verbal language cues can be an important diagnostic tool for an observant health professional. Patients may use their hands to describe types of pain, and the health professional must be attuned to such gestures as a form of non-verbal communication. For instance, for chest pain, a clenched fist conveys the gripping quality of the pain of cardiac ischaemia, while movement of the fingertips up and down the sternum may indicate oesophageal pain.[65] When supine patients present at an emergency room with crossed limbs (ankles crossed, hands crossed behind necks, folded hands over the upper abdomen), they are highly unlikely to have an acute condition.[66] Nurses who spend entire shifts with patients can get to read their facial expressions and their baseline affect, and determine when they are in pain, without words needing to be expressed.[67]

Developing expertise in interpreting non-verbal language allows a health care professional to glean an insight into the accuracy, or otherwise, of people's words. Because of politeness, embarrassment, confusion, or a deliberate intent

Box 2.5: Activity 5

- Referring to the non-verbal stocktake (Table 2.2), which of those aspects would you consider have a positive or negative impact on communication?
- How can you explore your own values and beliefs regarding these non-verbal cues?
- What evidence do you have that your values and beliefs about non-verbal communications are accurate?

To answer this, you could also discuss the features from the non-verbal stocktake with a close friend or colleague from a different cultural background. Remember you are exploring your values, not constructing stereotypes.

- Now revisit Activity 2. What aspects of non-verbal language may have had an impact on the situation?

Table 2.2: Non-verbal stocktake[68]

Type of non-verbal communication	*Non-verbal cues*
Physical appearance	race, gender, clothing, colour of clothing, grooming, body shape/size
Eye contact	direct, indirect, gazing, staring
Facial expressions	smiling, frowning, raised eyebrows, crying, laughing
Vocal cues	pitch, pace, volume, rhythm, silence, pause, tone, speech errors, responsiveness, pronunciation
Body language	hand and arm gestures, fidgeting, head movements, foot and leg movements
Posture	standing, sitting, relaxed, stiff, stooped
Proximity	use of space, physical distance between communicators
Touch	handshake, pat, physical contact during physical examinations
Time usage	early, late, on time, overtime, rushed, slow to respond
Environment	setting , furniture placement, lighting, temperature, colour

to deceive, patients sometimes say things that do not fully express their true feelings, and may even contradict them.

Sign language

Sign language, as used by people with hearing and speech impairment, is a visual representation of language. The signed symbols depict objects, concepts, and feelings.[69] Because signing is symbolic and not literal, there are hundreds of different sign languages spoken throughout the world. The variety and complexity of these languages present a challenge to the health professional. This awareness can aid in the sensitive choice of interpreters and the use of some simple strategies to enhance communication. As empirical studies have shown, the absence of sign language interpreters in medical settings causes much distress for individual deaf patients as well as diminishing the health of the whole deaf community.[70]

However, some deaf people may refuse to use an interpreter. Fox recounts a tale of one such woman, who had suffered headaches for more than forty years, but did not want to use an interpreter when consulting with a doctor.[71] Communication had proved difficult, if not impossible, with consultations with several specialists over the years. On a later visit, Fox attempted to communicate through the written word and diagrams, and was able to successfully diagnose and treat the woman. He made the point that he should not have assumed her deafness and ability to speak meant she could not write either. Chilton, however, considers the use of written notes, as well as lip reading and the use of unqualified interpreters, as ineffective.[72] This would be especially true when provider and patient do not share a common language.

The principles involved with working with a sign interpreter are much the same as working with other language interpreters, although the technique differs. The sign interpreter should sit beside and slightly behind the person conducting the interview (but not so as to be obscured by the bright light from a window), so the patient can see both easily. Adequate lighting is essential.[73]

CONCLUSION

In this chapter, we have seen how language is informed by a complex interrelationship of culture, the written, the spoken, and the non-verbal, (including sign) language. The use of language is therefore dependent on context, and an awareness of the language and expressions that we use during an interaction is the key to open communication. Without open communication, difficulties may be encountered in patient/user compliance and positive treatment outcomes.

Language is also a key to fully informed consent. How can a patient be truly informed without complete information? Similarly, how can a patient participate meaningfully in personal care decisions without adequate information, which can be provided through interpreters or bilingual health workers? This, as Woloshin et al. point out, violates patient autonomy.[74] Since patient autonomy is a fundamental component of Western medical decision-making and practice, adequate communication transpires as a prerequisite of ethical practice. These issues are explored further by Catherine Berglund in Chapter 8 in which the interaction and exchange of information between professional and patient is the focus of discussion on informed decision-making.

NOTES

1 Hadley, A. (1993). *Teaching Language in Context.* Heinle & Heinle, Boston, p. 357.

2 Woloshin, S., Bickell, N.A., Schwartz, L.M., Gany, F. & Welch, H.G. (1995). Language barriers in medicine in the United States. *Journal of the American Medical Association*, 273, 9, pp. 724–8, p. 724.

3 Godbey, S.F. & George, S. (1997). Getting the facts: Doctor, doctor, gimme the news. *Prevention*, 49, 2, pp. 30–2.

4 Coulter, A., Entwistle, V. & Gilbert, D. (1999). Sharing decisions with patients: Is the information good enough? *British Medical Journal*, 318, 7179, pp. 318–22.

5 Lee Zoreda, M. (1997). Cross-cultural relations and pedagogy. *American Behavioral Scientist*, 40, 7, pp. 923–35.

6 Buttjes, D. (1991). Mediating languages and cultures: The social and intercultural dimension restored, in D. Buttjes & M. Byram (eds) *Mediating Languages and Cultures: Towards an Intercultural Theory of Foreign Language Education.* Multicultural Matters, Clevedon, p. 7.

7 Faulkner, A. (1998). ABC of palliative care: Communication with patients, families, and other professionals. *British Medical Journal,* 316, 7125, pp. 130–2.

8 Weinger, M.B. & England, C.E. (1990). Ergonomic and human factors affecting anesthetic vigilance and monitoring performance in the operating room environment. *Anesthesiology,* 73, p. 995.

9 Coulter et al., 1999.

10 Maher, L. (1998). Motivational interviewing: What, when, and why? *Patient Care,* 32, 14, p. 55.

11 Woloshin et al., 1995.

12 Stewart, M.A. (1995). Effective physician-patient communication and health outcomes: A review. *Canadian Medical Association Journal,* 152, pp. 1423–33.

13 Leopold, N., Cooper, J. & Clancy, C. (1996). Sustained partnership in primary care. *Journal of Family Care,* 2, pp. 129–7.

14 Trentholm, S. & Jensen, A. (1992). *Interpersonal Communication,* 2nd ed. Wadsworth, Belmont, Cal.

15 Woloshin et al., 1995.

16 San Jose Hospital Family Practice Residency Program [SJHFPRP] (1994). Five vignettes of cross-cultural care. *Patient Care,* 28, 11, pp. 120–3.

17 Wilson, S. & Billones, H. (1994). The Filipino elder: Implications for nursing practice. *Journal of Gerontological Nursing,* 20, 8, pp. 31–6.

18 O'Hara, E.M. & Zhan, L. (1994). Cultural and pharmacological considerations when caring for Chinese elders. *Journal of Gerontological Nursing,* 20, 10, pp. 11–16.

19 SJHFPRP, 1994.

20 Buchwald, D., Caralis, P.V., Gany, F., Hardt, E.J., Johnson, T.M., Muecke, M.A. & Putsch, R.W. (1994). Caring for patients in a multicultural society. *Patient Care,* 28, 11, pp. 105–10.

21 SJHFPRP, 1994.

22 SJHFPRP, 1994.

23 Hudgings, D.W. (1995). The curse. *Journal of Family Practice,* 41, p. 408.

24 Buchwald et al., 1994.

25 Benner, P. (1984). *From Novice to Expert.* Addison-Wesley, Menlo Park, Calif.

26 Skelton, J.R. & Hobbs, F.D.R. (1999). Concordancing: Use of language-based research in medical communication. *Lancet,* 353, 91147, pp. 108–11.

27 Faulkner, 1998.

28 Ptacek, J.T. & Eberhardt, T.L. (1996). Breaking bad news: A review of the literature. *Journal of the American Medical Association,* 276, 6, pp. 496–502.

29 Platt, F.W. (1994). I hope I answered your questions all right. *Patient Care,* 28, 19, p. 88.

30 Fu, D. & Townsend, J.S. (1998). Cross-cultural dilemmas in writing: Need for transformation in teaching and learning. *College Teaching,* Fall, p. 128.

31 Naish, J., Brown J. & Denton, B. (1994). Intercultural consultations: Investigation of factors that deter non-English-speaking women from attending their general practitioners for cervical screening. *British Medical Journal*, 309, 6962, pp. 1126–8.
32 Rafuse, J. (1993). Multicultural medicine: 'Dealing with a population you weren't quite prepared for'. *Canadian Medical Association Journal*, 148, 2, pp. 282–5.
33 Prince, D. & Nelson, M. (1995). Teaching Spanish to emergency medicine residents. *Academy of Emergency Medicine*, 2, pp. 32–7.
34 Woloshin et al., 1995.
35 Phelan, M. & Parkman, S. (1995). How to do it: Work with an interpreter. *British Medical Journal*, 311, 7004, pp. 555–7.
36 Phelan & Parkman, 1995.
37 Chussil, J.T. (1998). Cultural competency in nursing. *Dermatology Nursing*, 10, 6, p. 393.
38 Chussil, 1998.
39 Phelan & Parkman, 1995.
40 Ebden, P., Carey, O.J., Bhatt, A. & Harrison, B. (1988). The bilingual consultation. *Lancet*, 1 (8581), p. 347.
41 Breen, L.M. (1999). What should I do if my patient does not speak English? *Journal of the American Medical Association*, 282, 9, p. 819.
42 Phelan & Parkman, 1995, p. 555.
43 Buchwald, D., Caralis, P.V., Gany, F., Hardt, E.J., Muecke, M.A. & Putsch, R.W. (1993). The medical interview across cultures. *Patient Care*, 27, 7, pp. 141–51.
44 Jones, D. & Gill, P. (1998). Breaking down language barriers: The NHS needs to provide accessible interpreting services for all. *British Medical Journal*, 316, 7143, p. 1476.
45 Phelan & Parkman, 1995.
46 Phelan & Parkman, 1995.
47 Phelan & Parkman, 1995.
48 Phelan & Parkman, 1995.
49 Mohan, T., McGregor, H., Saunders, S. & Archee, R. (1997). *Communicating! Theory and Practice*. 4th edn, Harcourt Brace, Sydney, p. 33.
50 Williams, M.V., Parker, R.M., Baker, D.W., Parikh, N.S., Pitkin, K., Coates, W.C. & Nurss, J.R. (1995). Inadequate functional health literacy among patients at two public hospitals. *Journal of the American Medical Association*, 274, no. 21, pp. 1677–82.
51 Kefalides, P.T. (1999). Illiteracy: The silent barrier to health care. *Annals of Internal Medicine*, 130, 4, pp. 333–6.
52 Gunning, R. (1968). *The Technique of Clear Writing*. McGraw-Hill, New York.
53 Pallen, M. (1995). Guide to the Internet: Electronic mail. *British Medical Journal*, 311, 7018, pp. 1487–90.
54 Brailer, D.J. & Hackett, T.S. (1997). Points (and clicks) on quality. *Hospital Health Networks*, 71, 22, p. 32; Ferguson, T. (1997). Health care in cyberspace: Patients lead the revolution. *Futurist*, 31, 6, p. 29.
55 Spielberg, A.R. (1998). On call and online: Sociohistorical, legal, and ethical implications of e-mail for the patient–physician relationship. *Journal of the American Medical Association*, 280, 15, p. 1353.

56 Green, L. (1996). A better way to keep in touch with patients: Electronic mail. *Medical Economics*, 73, p. 153.

57 Pallen, 1995.

58 Seifert, P.C. (1999). Communication—Speaking, surfing, and smiling. *Association of Operating Room Nurses Journal*, 70, 4, pp. 558, 561.

59 Knapp, M. L. (1980). *Essentials of Non Verbal Communication.* Holt, Rinehart & Winston, New York.

60 Brown, T. (1997). Body talk. *Nursing Standard*, 11, 30, pp. 21–3.

61 Brown, 1997.

62 Rieman, D. (1986). Noncaring and caring in the clinical setting: Patients' descriptions. *Topics in Clinical Nursing*, 8, 2, pp. 30–6.

63 Drew, N. (1986). Exclusion and confirmation: A phenomenology of patients' experiences with caregivers. *IMAGE: A Journal of Nursing Scholarship*, 18, 2, pp. 39–43.

64 Brown, 1997.

65 Edmondstone, W.M. (1995). Cardiac chest pain: Does body language help the diagnosis? *British Medical Journal*, 311, 7021, pp. 1660–1.

66 Rapoport, M.J., Leonov, Y. & Leibowitz, A. (1995). Body language in the emergency room. *Lancet*, 345, 8956, p. 1060.

67 See, for example, Peterson, A.B. & Hall, T. (1999). Nursing challenge: Caring for a patient with complex, multiple complications. *Heart and Lung: The Journal of Acute and Critical Care*, 28, 5, pp. 373–6.

68 Silverman, J., Kurtz, S. & Draper, J. (1998). *Skills for Communicating with Patients.* Radcliffe Medical Press, Oxford, p. 75.

69 Finegan, E., Besnier, N., Blair, D. & Collins, P. (1997). *Language: Its Structure and Use.* 2nd edn, Harcourt Brace, Sydney, p. 26.

70 Chilton, E.E. (1996). Ensuring effective communication: The duty of health care providers to supply sign language interpreters for deaf patients. *Hastings Law Journal*, 47, 3, p. 871.

71 Fox, N. (1999). A memorable patient: A communication headache. *British Medical Journal*, 318, 71186, p. 802.

72 Chilton, 1996.

73 Phelan & Parkman, 1995.

74 Woloshin et al., 1995.

3

Listening

Jill Gordon

> It is the disease of not listening, the malady of not marking, that I am troubled withal.
>
> Falstaff[1]

This chapter is about listening to patients, their families, and other health care professionals. Listening skills in history taking are examined, and the process of history taking becomes a case study in communication. Listening to insights offered by other treating practitioners (of all disciplines) or fellow professionals is also discussed. Active listening is the first step to understanding and starting on the assessment and treatment process.

LISTENING AS A STARTING POINT FOR COMMUNICATION

Listening is a key component of information gathering. Sometimes the process of listening begins before the patient and doctor meet, since patients may have reputations that precede them, health professionals who know them well, or family members who wish to provide information prior to a first contact. The term 'doctor' is used here because it is shorter than 'health care professional' and less clumsy than acronyms such as HCP. However, the reader may wish to insert another type of health care professional here; the message will be essentially the same.

The words that patients use at the beginning, as at the end, of a clinical encounter are often especially interesting and relevant to the problems that they bring. When a woman's husband arrived late for a joint consultation, her first statement on entering the consulting room was *'He's never there when you need him most'*, and indeed that problem had always lain at the heart of their relationship difficulties.

While such statements often occur outside the formal consultation and outside the consulting space, they can all be viewed as integral to the communication process.

Despite its diagnostic value, doctors often prevent their patients from completing this critically important opening statement.[2, 3] In Beckman and Frankel's 1984 study, patients consulting doctors (81 per cent of whom were residents in internal medicine) were given the opportunity to finish their first statement in only 23 per cent of cases. Doctors' interruptions appear to be innocuous enough; they are mostly questions for **clarification**, or specific closed questions, but the questions tend to have the effect of redirecting the consultation.[4] One might wish to defend the doctors in this study on the grounds that they were listening closely and simply needed to know more about the patient's problem in order to understand it better. However, interruptions made during the critical opening phase of a consultation resulted in patients providing less information overall. The interruptions were found to be associated with late-arising problems that might have been brought forward earlier, had the doctors remained attentively silent. In addition, the doctors' questions, instead of facilitating the consultations, actually led to the doctors taking over the consultation in 94 per cent of instances. Only one interruption out of 52 was followed by the opportunity for the patient to return to their own agenda. Interruptions at the beginning of a consultation appeared to make patients less confident that they would be able to choose the issues that were troubling them, and more likely to allow the doctors to dictate which issues to pursue and which to ignore.

The answer to many of these problems in opening the consultation can be found in the technique of using '**wait time**'. Waiting longer than would feel comfortable in an ordinary conversation offers powerful encouragement for patients to continue to describe their concerns. After waiting until a natural break occurs, the doctor can add a question such as *'and is there anything else that is worrying you?'* This additional encouragement conveys the information that the patient is not limited to a single concern and often results in other major concerns being expressed.

LISTENING AS THE CONSULTATION PROGRESSES

Why might doctors spend more time speaking than listening? Do they believe that early interruptions will reduce the amount of time that a consultation might otherwise require? Do they believe that patients expect them to dominate the consultation? Do they think that 'conversational' speech, with the normal interruptions that we all tend to make, is more appropriate than attentive silence?

The evidence suggests that these beliefs are misguided. Marvel et al. found that patients who were allowed to complete their concerns used an average of only 32 seconds to do so, compared with 26 seconds before interruption occurred. Early redirection is also associated with late arising concerns, which consume more time towards the end of the consultation.[5]

The habit of dominating consultations has become less acceptable to consumers who now seek a more equal partnership in their pursuit of health. Studies of consultation behaviour also make clear that consultations are not conversations, but skilled technical manoeuvres that are part of the diagnostic process. Listening is, in this respect, part of both the science and the art of medicine. In a 'normal' conversation, individuals expect to contribute to the discussion on a more or less equal basis. In fact it is easy to observe that many 'normal' conversations are characterised less by listening than by waiting to speak. Consultations are not debates, and a consultation in which the doctor says only as much as is strictly necessary during the information-gathering phase is likely to yield more relevant and valuable information.

Goldberg et al. found that doctors who demonstrate that they are listening, with good eye contact, relaxed posture, minimal encouragers and withholding information in the early stages of the consultation, are better able to identify signs of emotional distress.[6] Davenport et al. found that these behaviours lead to patients providing doctors with more information.[7] One of the interesting characteristics of doctors who elicit more information is good timing, that is the ability to balance listening and other behaviours such as asking directive or closed questions. Golberg and Huxley have described a series of four filters that help to determine whether or not patients with common mental disorders will be admitted to hospital.[8] The first filter is the patient's own illness behaviour. The second is the ability of the care-giver to detect disorder. The third and fourth are respectively, referral to a mental health service and admission to hospital. The second filter, when the doctor–patient encounter occurs, is the one in which active listening is a critical determinant of care from that point onwards.

As well as listening to the patient's words, listening to the tone, speed, volume, and steadiness of the voice is important. Patients are more likely to offer these cues to doctors who listen well.[9] While strong emotional states may be obvious from the patient's behaviour, more subtle variations may not be evident except in vocal changes. Is the tone tentative, irritable, aggressive, or angry? Is it wheedling or obsequious? Is speech slow, accelerated, or highly circumstantial? Does the patient speak softly or loudly? Is there a vocal tremor or any form of dysarthria? Some aphasic disorders develop slowly and can be missed or attributed to psychological factors unless subtle changes are picked up by the careful listener. A range of diagnostic possibilities can be suggested by alterations in speech, and changes may only be evident when patient and doctor are familiar with each other. For example, the difference between a patient's normal speech and speech during an episode of mild depression may not be evident to a person who does not know what 'normal' speech is for this person.

Patients usually bring more than one problem into the consultation.[10] Listening carefully throughout the consultation reduces the likelihood of redirecting the patient towards one specific complaint at the expense of other concerns. Leaving enough time at the end of the consultation allows the doctor to listen to any last minute concerns, although these final words are fewer if the listening task has been done well in the early stages of the consultation.

LISTENING AND OBSERVATION

The doctor's instinctive reaction to different verbal presentations can contribute valuable information, especially when there is a 'fit' between what is heard and what is seen. A well-dressed, attractive patient may create a visual impression that leads the doctor to overestimate his or her intelligence. The reverse also applies. Listening carefully to the patient's own words can be a more accurate indicator of how well the details of the diagnosis and management plan are understood than reliance on appearances.

Inconsistencies between what is seen and heard can also provide insight into the patient's coping skills. When the psychological mechanism being used is denial, the patient usually maintains reasonable congruency between what is said, how it is said and the accompanying non-verbal behaviours. However, the doctor may be struck by unreasonably optimistic expectations on the patient's part. When patients are simply trying to hide feelings of which they are aware, it may be easier for the doctor to notice the discrepancy and for patients to admit their concerns.

The **Johari Window** has been used to illustrate four states of awareness that underpin human relationships.[11] The clinical task is to discover and manage significant facts about the patient's health status, a task that can only be achieved if the doctor listens well. It is likely that some elements of any patient's health status will be unknown from time to time (Quadrant 4) but an ideal professional relationship, one that is likely to maximise health benefits, can be represented by Quadrant 1. In this quadrant the patient's own insights into his or her health are aligned with those of the doctor. Sometimes patients will deliberately withhold information from the doctor (Quadrant 3) and in this situation, acutely tuned

	Known to self	*Not known to self*
Known to doctor	1 OPEN	2 BLIND
Not known to doctor	3 HIDDEN	4 UNKNOWN

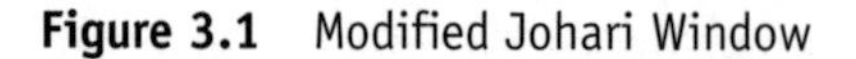
Figure 3.1 Modified Johari Window

listening skills are vital. In Quadrant 2, the doctor is aware of information that the patient does not know. This situation is represented by that stage of the diagnostic process in which a doctor receives information from the history, physical examination, or investigations that have not yet been transmitted to the patient. This stage occurs and recurs throughout the clinical relationship, and is the main reason why patients seek the help of health professionals, that is, to uncover important information about their health. Listening is one of major skills of the diagnostic process.

A common situation in everyday consultations occurs when a patient fears the possibility of a serious diagnosis, but also fears that they will look foolish or hypochondriacal if they ask the doctor whether their cough, headache, or abdominal pain might have serious implications. Because of this ambivalence, it is often possible to pick up a hesitancy of tone or a note of false bravado, depending on the patient's personality. Reflecting back to the patient the tone of concern, or the worried look not only leads to a more accurate appraisal of the patient's emotional state, but it also demonstrates how carefully the doctor is attending to what is being said. This is almost certainly the reason why patients reveal more to doctors who are good 'detectors' of emotional disturbance, that is, who operate comfortably in Quadrant 2.[12]

Listening therefore provides both useful information and appropriate reassurance. Patients frequently and justifiably fear that they will not be able to make the doctor listen and understand; that they will not be able to prevent the doctor from jumping to hasty conclusions. Words of reassurance, particularly if offered prematurely, can work against the therapeutic process.[13] Patients do not expect facile responses, but evidence of the doctor's expertise, demonstrated through a careful history and examination and the ability to explain clearly what has been found and what can be done to manage the problem.

LISTENING AND CLARIFYING

Although **minimal encouragers** are the most effective method for eliciting the patient's concerns at the beginning of a consultation, clarification is usually essential as the consultation progresses. Clarification demonstrates that the doctor is attending to what is being said, helps patients to be more precise about their symptoms, avoids ambiguity and encourages them to elaborate on elements of particular interest to the doctor. Listening and observing serve as the foundation for clarification for both doctor and patient. For the doctor, listening combined with observation provides the starting point for accurate diagnosis and appropriate management. Remembering items of information from past consultations allows the doctor to demonstrate that what has been said has been carefully listened to, and provides the patient with further evidence that the doctor will integrate relevant information as needed. For patients, attentive listening provides reassurance that their concerns are being taken seriously. This generates trust that enables patients to bring forward more details that might otherwise embarrass or frighten them.

LISTENING AS A THERAPEUTIC INTERVENTION

The therapeutic importance of listening is clear in the various forms of psychotherapy for which listening is the mainstay. It has been exploited by alternative or complementary medicine.[14] However, listening is part of every clinical interaction.[15] It is the basis for accurate reassurance when nothing seriously wrong can be found, and it is the basis for reassurance that help is at hand. It is particularly important when no further medical intervention is possible. In the field of palliative care, Maguire has demonstrated some of the problems that health care professionals experience when it comes to dealing with dying patients.[16] In one study, patients were found to be highly selective in what they disclosed to nursing staff, showing a strong bias towards disclosing physical symptoms. Concerns about the future, their appearance during the illness, and their loss of independence were withheld more than 80 per cent of the time.[17] Patients make their own judgments about what doctors, nurses, and other health professionals can bear, just as they choose to withhold information from family and friends. The capacity to listen empathically to all of a patient's concerns, but particularly to concerns about death and dying, is a powerful therapeutic intervention.

There are four key aspects of human experience that give rise to most of the concerns that humanity shares. Irvin Yalom summarises them as four 'givens': '*the inevitability of death for each of us and for those we love, the freedom to make our lives as we will, our ultimate aloneness and, finally, the absence of any obvious meaning or sense to life*'.[18] Because of their fundamental importance, it is possible to listen for the words that patients typically use to express issues of deep concern. Expressions of concern about unexplained symptoms or compromised function foreshadow their fear of death. Whenever patients use words like 'choices' and 'decision' they are acknowledging the dangerous side of free choice, and are usually seeking expert advice and support. 'Aloneness' is never more acutely felt than when a diagnosis of serious illness seems possible. Children may express their aloneness as unexplained tummy pains or a refusal to go to school. Adolescents may express it by the parsimony of their language when dealing with health professionals whose ability for genuine empathy they doubt. Finally, questions about the meaning of life become increasingly significant with the passage of time or when a serious illness occurs. Even patients who have a deep religious conviction may find themselves questioning the security of their place in the world. Inevitably the careful listener recognises one, but usually more of the words that convey these fundamental concerns in all but the briefest consultations.

The therapeutic benefits of listening are available to both patient and doctor. Listening to patients' deepest concerns is a great privilege. Patients' stories arise out of a range of experiences that may have included wartime experiences, deprivation, suffering, loss and grief, courage, and achievement. Careful listening enables the attentive doctor to benefit personally and also to act as a faithful witness, carrying information from one patient to another. A patient who has survived a difficult illness and who has found a way of coping can benefit another patient via the doctor who tells the second patient (with due regard for confidentiality) a little about the experiences of the first. Doctors probably rank second only to family members as recipients of this experience and understanding.

Doctors also derive important but less uplifting insights by listening to patients' stories of greed, jealousy, intimidation, anger, manipulation, sadness, and helplessness. Listening can be a life-saving skill if it enables the doctor to detect the situations in which a patient's reference to suicide or violent intent is more than an expression of extreme emotion without intent.

PROBLEMS WITH LISTENING

Listening can be compromised by the listener's fatigue, by denial, by prejudice, by the repetitious complaints of the hypochondriac, by the challenge of confronting the difficult patient with some truths and by the doctor's own personal worries, particularly if they are similar to the patient's.

Although some of these problems are inevitable at times, there exists an ethical obligation to approach the consultation fully prepared to devote attention to the patient's concerns. This may mean careful attention to the daily and weekly schedule in order to provide sufficient time for each consultation and for breaks. In the public health system, the doctor's control over pressures in the workplace may be limited, but some doctors nevertheless convey to patients respect and attentive listening, even when time is very limited. In the sphere of privately funded health care, fear of losing patients, personal greed or unrealistic expectations of how much consulting can be done within a certain time-frame, are chiefly responsible for setting up situations in which the doctor is too busy to listen properly. In both the public and the private system, acquiring the emotional maturity to listen well is the doctor's greatest personal challenge.

'If your only tool is a hammer, everything looks like a nail.'[19] The listening doctor's knowledge base influences what is heard and how that information is interpreted. Personal prejudices are also relevant. Women, who constitute a larger proportion of ambulatory patients, are particularly likely to be perceived as '**heartsink**' patients.[20] Doctors who characterise more of their patients as

causing a heartsink reaction were found to have lower job satisfaction, lack of training in communication skills and a greater perceived workload.[21]

An example of this danger posed by bias can be illustrated by the experience of the gynaecologist who was consulted for the first time by a woman aged 50 who complained of headache and depression. The gynaecologist attributed these symptoms to the menopause. Six months later the woman died from a brain tumour that could have been diagnosed and treated if the gynaecologist had examined her fundi, noted the marked papilloedema and referred her to a neurosurgeon. The gynaecologist's listening ear was attuned to a limited number of histories. Had the woman consulted a neurosurgeon, his or her familiarity with this presentation could have led to immediate diagnosis and treatment. The fact that in some countries such as the USA gynaecologists operate as primary care providers increases the possibility of premature closure on such symptoms—the hammer and nail problem. Listening must be accompanied by an active inner process of questioning, hypothesis generation, sifting, differential diagnosis, and hypothesis testing. Premature closure can have tragic consequences.

Other problems with listening include the competing needs to feel in control, to impress, and to transmit important information. Understanding that there are limits to patients' ability to absorb information at any particular time can result in a better balance between listening and informing.

LISTENING TO FAMILY AND TO OTHER PROFESSIONALS

Listening to people other than the patient can facilitate understanding of the patient's problem, but it will inevitably introduce an element of bias. The advantages of obtaining such information should clearly outweigh this inevitable disadvantage. Preconceptions about the nature of the clinical problem, including preconceptions gleaned from other health care professionals, can compromise accurate diagnosis. It is important to balance the value of listening to others against the value of forming one's own view, based on the patient's own story.

Listening to the contribution of patients' family members requires special listening skills. Anxiety may lead family members to exaggerate symptoms in order to ensure that their parent, spouse, or child receives prompt and sympathetic attention. On the other hand, family members find it extremely frustrating to have their input discounted. The axiom in paediatrics is that *'every mother is a world expert in her own children'* and there can be no justification for ignoring the information that parents bring.

Listening to insights offered by other treating practitioners of all disciplines or by fellow professionals can be extremely helpful, since every observation is filtered by our own biases. These same biases can make it difficult to accept the advice of colleagues, and taking the time and effort to explore the reasons for such reluctance can lead to particularly valuable insights. Asking oneself why one finds it difficult to consider certain opinions voiced by other professionals can yield valuable self-knowledge. Nursing staff often find it frustrating when doctors appear not to listen to their opinions,[22] and women working within any occupational group are aware that they are less likely to be 'heard' than men.

LISTENING IN DIFFERENT ENVIRONMENTS

The emergency room, home visits, and crowded wards all pose different challenges for the listener. In each case there can be considerable distractions. Whenever possible, distracting features of the environment should be removed. These may include visual distractions, family members, and excessive noise levels. Even the act of drawing curtains around a bed can enable the listener to hear the patient more easily, even when the noise level remains the same. Wherever possible a quiet space should be used. Television and radio turned off for the duration of the interview. If circumstances permit, it may be better to obtain a brief history and return later in the hope of fewer distractions. When this is not possible, documenting the context may be an important element of the medical record, making it clear that the circumstances, being less than ideal, may have compromised the doctor's opportunity to listen to the patient's story.

One special context for listening occurs when both patient and doctor know that the patient has a serious illness. Maguire et al. have shown how hard it is to maintain a listening attitude at this time.[23] The doctor's psychological adjustment is important,[24] and this underlines the need for professional care-givers to attend to their own emotional well-being before they can be free to listen openly to their patients.

CAN LISTENING SKILLS BE TAUGHT?

Listening skills are only one of the communication skills that can be taught.[25] An attentive posture, lack of hurry, appropriate eye contact, and minimal encouragers all contribute to the listening state.

A simple method to prevent precipitate action is taught to beginning parachutists: take a breath and repeat the words *'Not now, but now'* before pulling the cord. Medical students and inexperienced doctors can apply this rule in order to achieve an appropriate 'wait time', especially in the early stages of a consultation. Audiotapes and videotapes of consultations can be used to find out whether or not patients are being interrupted or redirected during consultations.

Recognising the key words that refer, directly or indirectly, to death, key decisions, loneliness, or questioning the meaning or significance of illness can unearth a rich lode in the search for better understanding of each patient's individual concerns and the significance of their individual experiences.[26] Again, tape recording can be valuable as a means for reviewing consultations for messages that may have been missed.[27] These supporting activities can help the clinician to maintain the habit of **reflection** that is critical to the development of finely tuned listening skills.[28]

NOTES

1 Shakespeare, W. (1925). *King Henry IV*, in T. Donovan (ed.), *The Falstaff Plays of William Shakespeare.* Sydney: Angus & Robertson.

2 Beckman, H.B. and Frankel, R.M. (1984). The effect of physician behavior on the collection of data, *Annals of Internal Medicine*, 101: pp. 692–6.

3 Suchman, A.L., Markakis, K., Beckman, H.B. and Frankel, R. (1997). A model of empathic communication in the medical interview, *Journal of the American Medical Association*, 277: pp. 678–82.

4 Beckman, H.B. and Frankel, R.M. 1984.

5 Marvel, M.K., Epstein, R.M., Flowers, K. and Beckman, H.B. (1999). Soliciting the patient's agenda: have we improved? *Journal of the American Medical Association,* 281: pp. 283–7.

6 Goldberg, D.P., Jenkins, L., Millar, T. and Faragher, E.B. (1993). The ability of trainee general practitioners to identify emotional distress among their patients, *Psychological Medicine*, 23: pp. 185–93.

7 Davenport, S., Goldberg, D. and Millar, T. (1987). How psychiatric disorders are missed during medical consultations, *Lancet,* 3: pp. 439–42.

8 Goldberg, D. and Huxley, P. (1992). *Common Mental Disorders.* London: Routledge.

9 Stewart, M. and Roter, D. (eds), (1989). *Communicating with Medical Patients.* Newbury Park, Cal., Sage Publications.

10 Stewart, M. and Roter, D. (eds), 1989.

11 Luft, J. and Ingham, H. (1955). The Johari Window, a graphic model of interpersonal awareness, *Proceedings of the Western Training Laboratory in Group Development.* Los Angeles, University of California.

12 Goldberg, D. and Huxley, P. 1992.

13 Maguire, P., Faulkner, A., Booth, K., Elliott, C. and Hillier, V. (1996). Helping cancer patients disclose their concerns, *European Journal of Cancer,* 32: pp. 78–81.

14 Coulehan, J. (1999). An alternative view: listening to patients, *Lancet*, 354: pp. 1467–8.

15 Cassell, E. (1999). Diagnosing suffering: a perspective, *Annals of Internal Medicine*, 131: 531–4.

16 Maguire, P. (1998). Breaking bad news, *European Journal of Surgical Oncology*, 24: pp. 188–91.

17 Heaven, C.M. and Maguire, P. (1997). Disclosure of concerns by hospice patients and their identification by nurses, *Palliative Medicine*, 11: pp. 283–90.

18 Yalom, I. (1989). *Love's Executioner*. London: Bloomsbury, p. 4.

19 Japanese proverb.

20 O'Dowd, T.C. (1988). Five years of heartsink patients in general practice, *British Journal of Medicine*, 297: pp. 528–30.

21 Mathers, N., Jones, N. and Hannay, D. (1995). Heartsink patients: a study of their general practitioners, *British Journal of General Practice*, 45: pp. 293–6.

22 Pringle, R. (1998). *Sex and Medicine: Gender, Power and Authority in the Medical Profession*. Melbourne: Cambridge University Press.

23 Maguire, P. et al. 1996.

24 Vaillant, G.C. and Sobowale, N. (1972). Some psychological vulnerabilities of physicians: a review, *Comprehensive Psychiatry*, 15: pp. 519–30.

25 Maguire, P. (1990). Can communication skills be taught? *British Journal of Hospital Medicine*, 43: pp. 215–16.

26 Smith, R.C., Hoppe, R.B. (1991). The patient's story: integrating the patient- and physician-centered approaches to interviewing. *Annals of Internal Medicine*, 115: pp. 470–7.

27 Maguire, P., Roe, P., Goldberg, D., Jones, S., Hyde, C., O'Dowd, T. (1978). The value of feedback in teaching interviewing skills to medical students, *Psychological Medicine*, 8: pp. 695–704.

28 Schön, D.A. (1987). *Educating the Reflective Practitioner: Toward a New Design for Teaching and Learning in the Professions*. San Francisco: Jossey-Bass.

4

Questioning

Dimity Pond

Clinical practice often requires the use of questioning. Some practitioners may view this as a relatively simple skill associated with history taking, with more complex skills being required for diagnosis and management. However, questioning may be used at all stages of the clinical process: for history taking, diagnosis, and management. Experienced practitioners may use questioning in subtle and interesting ways to deepen their understanding of patients and their problems. The form of questioning and the uses to which it is put may transmit to the respondent a model of interaction in which they have little power, or it may transmit a model in which they are the centre of the interaction. What follows is a brief review of this important and interesting mode of interaction in the context of a clinical interview.

WHAT IS QUESTIONING?

Questioning has been defined as a request for information, whether factual or otherwise.[1] Such requests may occur at all levels of social interaction, from the very earliest communication of a small child to the most structured and sophisticated settings of adult working life. The questioning discussed in the rest of this chapter is that used in clinical settings, whether it is doctor–patient interactions, counselling settings, or the work of other health professionals in caring for people.

Even in this limited context, questioning may take many different forms, and fulfil a variety of functions. In the following discussion, the functions identified are those important to the clinician: history taking, diagnosis, and management of the problem. In addition, questioning and the form that it takes help to establish the nature of the relationship between a practitioner and a respondent. This relationship may be therapeutic, or it may impede therapy. This chapter therefore includes a discussion of the use of questions in influencing the interview process itself.

Some of the functions of questions connected with history taking and diagnosis are as follows:

- to obtain information
- to diagnose specific difficulties a respondent may have
- to ascertain the attitudes, feelings, and opinions of the respondent.

Other functions are more relevant to management:

- to assess the extent of the respondent's knowledge
- to encourage critical thought and evaluation.

However, others may be more relevant to the process of the clinical interaction:

- to maintain control of the interaction
- to express an interest in the respondent
- to encourage maximum participation by the respondent.

What types of questions work best for different functions?

A variety of classifications of questions have been proposed, including classification by function as above,[2] by the form of the question (e.g. verbal and non-verbal) and by the type of response required (e.g. division into closed and open).[3] The following discussion will focus on the types of questions best suited to the various functions of the clinical interview.

The most basic distinction in question form is between verbal and non-verbal questioning. Non-verbal questioning may include questions indicated by bodily movements (gestures, movements, facial expressions, eye behaviour, and posture), touching behaviour and paralanguage. Even the questions put in a clinical interview may be non-verbal—the raise of an eyebrow, a questioning look. These may encourage the respondent to continue their story. Questions may also use paralanguage (i.e. utterances that are not specifically words) in such settings. One example might be the use of a 'hmm-hunh?' after someone has made a statement, to encourage further elaboration of what they have been saying. Non-verbal behaviour may also impede an interview. Distracting finger tapping, checking of the watch, or even continuous writing may interfere with the respondent's answers.[4]

QUESTIONS THAT ASSIST HISTORY TAKING AND DIAGNOSIS

Questions that assist history-taking and diagnosis are questions that can be used to obtain information, diagnose specific difficulties, and ascertain attitudes, feelings, and opinions.

Closed and open questions

Closed questions usually begin with the words 'is', 'are', 'do', or 'did',[5] and require a short answer, often 'yes' or 'no'. For example, *'Are you troubled by a cough?'* or *'Is the cough dry or productive?'* **Open questions**, on the other hand, may begin with words such as 'what', 'how', 'why', 'could', or 'would',[6] and allow the respondent more freedom in deciding which answer to give. They also encourage the respondent to talk. An example might be: *'What has brought you here today?'* or *'Would you tell me a bit more about what is happening in the family at the moment?'*

Both these types of questions are useful for information gathering. In medical settings, open questions are often used initially (e.g. *'Why are you here today?'*), followed by more closed questions to clarify specific difficulties (e.g. *'Where exactly is the pain in your back?'*). Clearly, it is imperative that the respondent is allowed to identify the broad area of difficulty to the practitioner, and this can only be done by asking open questions first. As open questions encourage the respondent to talk, the practitioner may be able to use open questions early in the interview to identify not only the difficulty itself, but also some of the respondent's particular concerns, feelings, and ideas about it. This can be done quite quickly and simply by a few further enquiries, such as *'What part of this worries you most?'* and *'Could you tell me what your thoughts and feelings are about this?'* An understanding of the patient's ideas and concerns is helpful in formulating management strategies and in ensuring compliance.

This pattern of open questions followed by more specific closed questioning is called the 'open-to-closed cone'.[7] It can also be used with enquiries about specific symptoms. Most clinicians have a fairly clear understanding of the information they want about any particular symptom or series of symptoms. For instance, if a patient presents with pain, the practitioner will want to know about the nature of the pain (colicky, constant, sharp or dull, and so on), its site, radiation, precipitating and relieving factors, and accompanying symptoms. These features are often taught to students as a series of closed questions. It is possible to obtain much of this information by asking the patient an open question (e.g. *'Tell me about the pain'*), thus obtaining the patient's own version of the pain experience. The practitioner may then fill in missing information with a few closed questions. The advantage of this once again, is that the practitioner will glean an understanding of the patient's ideas and concerns as they tell their story. This is information that will be useful in the management phase.

In 1996, the Consumers' Health Forum, a peak health consumer body in Australia, commissioned a study of consumer views about quality in general practice. In the course of the study a series of nineteen group discussions were held with people independently recruited from the community. Discussions were audiotaped and subsequently analysed. The discussion groups members were encouraged to talk about their experiences with general practice. They were then asked to nominate attributes and issues that they felt were important to them in relation to general practice, and to rank these. Among the issues ranked with high priority and high frequency were interpersonal skills and qual-

Box 4.1

Doctor: Do you remember when the pain first came on? (Recall)
Patient: It was about three weeks ago, I think
Doctor: Were you doing anything in particular at the time? (Recall)
Patient: I'd just finished eating a Sunday roast
Doctor: Do you think the pain usually comes on after fatty meals like a roast? (Process)

ities of the general practitioner. A range of these attributes were identified, among them that consumers preferred a doctor who listens to, and responds carefully to, an individual patient's needs and circumstances.[8] Open questions facilitate this, and transmit to the respondent a sense that they are worthwhile and their story is worth listening to.

Recall and process questions

Another distinction that can be made is between questions that require the recall of simple information and questions that require the respondent to process information in a more complicated way before responding.[9] In a clinical interview simple recall questions may be used initially to establish some facts. This is often followed by more detailed questions that require the respondent to think harder about their answer. An example is given in Box 4.1.

Both recall and **process questions** can be used in history taking. Diagnosis, however, may require some assistance from the patient in terms of process questions. This is because diagnosis often requires the recognition of consistent patterns of symptoms, which may be identified by the patient once they are alerted to the issue by a process question.

Affective questions

Affective questions relate to attitudes and feelings of a respondent. They may be closed, open, recall, or process. Often, however, more open and more process questions will better elicit details in the affective domain. They are particularly relevant in a counselling setting, but are important in all types of consultation if a patient's concerns are to be addressed. Such questions convey a genuine sense of care and compassion, and a willingness to respond in depth to a patient's needs and concerns, characteristics that are highly valued by consumers.[10] Such questions may also assist with the practicalities of management, as demonstrated in Box 4.2.

Box 4.2

Doctor: Why have you stopped taking the tablets? (Open question)
Patient: I didn't really want to take them any more.
Doctor: Could you tell me a bit more about how you felt about taking the tablets? (Affective, open question)
Patient: I'm worried that they might be addictive, and my mother told me I should be able to get over this problem without tablets.

QUESTIONS THAT MAY ASSIST WITH PATIENT MANAGEMENT

Questions that may assist with patient management are questions that may be used to assess the extent of the respondent's knowledge, and to encourage critical thought and evaluation.

Probing questions

Probing questions are designed to encourage respondents to expand upon initial responses. There are a variety of types of **probing questions**: some are simply designed to encourage respondents to keep explaining, while others are more specific in their purpose. Some of the types are discussed below.

Non-verbal probes

At the beginning of this chapter, the use of non-verbal and paralanguage behaviour as questions was discussed. Often these behaviours indicate a simple desire for further information. Sometimes, however, a paraverbal or non-verbal cue may indicate surprise or incredulity, thus encouraging the respondent to justify themselves. Simply making eye contact with the patient may signal that they should continue. On the other hand, the clinician should be aware that non-verbal and paraverbal language may contradict the clinician's apparent desire to have questions answered. If the clinician looks at his watch, after asking a question, for example, this will signal that the answer is not really welcome, or should be constrained. The wearing of a badge of office (white coat or stethoscope) or the layout of the room (patient on the other side of a big desk) may also signal constraint, so that the patient will not respond to questions with all the relevant detail.

Justification probes

Sometimes verbal probes, such as the first question in Box 4.2, might create a need for justification. This is often helpful for a practitioner who wants to understand a patient's reasoning. However, the practitioner needs to be aware that justification probes may make a respondent defensive, and this may impede both the understanding necessary to improve management and the relationship inherent in the interaction.

Clarification probes

Clarification probes ask the respondent to clarify their response. Such questions may be used to assist the practitioner in understanding what a patient knows about their illness (e.g. *'You've mentioned that you may need different food when you exercise, tell me what you understand about the effect of exercise on your sugar levels?'*). This in turn can help the practitioner engage the patient in their own management, with improved understanding of the reasons for particular measures.

QUESTIONS THAT AFFECT THE PROCESS OF THE CLINICAL INTERACTION

These are questions that express an interest in the respondent, that encourage maximum participation, and that maintain control of the interaction.

The use of open questions

As described above, open questions are more likely to express an interest in the respondent and to encourage maximum participation. Respondents to an open question are more likely to feel that the questioner is interested in them. Such questions may also convey interest that is more than just clinical. Sometimes, a practitioner may use open questions of a social nature to indicate interest in the respondent (e.g. *'How's the family?'*). These questions may also provide valuable psychosocial background to enable the practitioner to better assess the patient.

The use of closed questions

Closed questions may be used as a means of closing off an overtalkative respondent.[11] A particularly useful way of doing this is to summarise what has been said and then ask if it is correct or not. This may be helpful as well towards the end of an interview, when time management is becoming an issue.

Leading questions

These questions are worded in such a way that respondents are led towards a desired response. While this may be necessary in a clinical scenario where time is limited, it is often detrimental to the interaction, as it mitigates against truthful responses. There are several types of leading questions:

- Conversational leads are often used to break the ice. An example might be *'Isn't it cold today?'*, expecting the answer *'Yes, it is'*.
- Simple leads exert a degree of pressure on the respondent to reply in a certain fashion. This can be counter-productive if a truthful response is wanted (e.g. *'Surely you never miss taking your contraceptive tablet?'*). However, some simple leads may actually give a respondent permission to be truthful (e.g. *'Can you tell me what drugs you haven't tried yet?'*).
- Implication leads are sometimes used to pass judgment on a patient (e.g. *'Did you know that what you are doing is very dangerous?'*). These, too, are often unhelpful, as they impede trust and honesty in the therapeutic relationship.
- Subtle leads are probably among the most common leading questions used in clinical practice. These questions are not obviously worded in a way to direct the questioner, but may nevertheless direct them. An example is the question *'Do you get headaches frequently, and if so, how often?'*.[12] The response to this question by forty subjects gave a mean headache frequency of 2.2 per week. When the question to a similar group of subjects was worded *'Do you get headaches occasionally, and if so, how often?'* they responded with a mean headache frequency of 0.7 per week. Subtle leads may indeed be so subtle that the practitioner may not recognise them!
- The tag question is a statement followed by a tag phrase that suggests how the respondent should answer. An example might be: *'You're happy to take the tablets, aren't you?'* It is very difficult to answer the tag 'aren't you' in the negative, so the respondent may feel coerced into stating a position that is not the case.

TRAPS FOR THE QUESTIONER

There are some other aspects of the clinical interaction that may make **questioning** less effective. A few of these traps are listed below. It is useful for practitioners to cultivate a reflective attitude towards questioning as well as other aspects of their practice. It may be that reflection on interviews that have not worked well, or indeed review of these by a peer or by videotape may alert practitioners to other aspects of questioning that may prove unhelpful.

Language

Practitioners should use language that is comprehensible to the respondent. This may be relatively easy when the respondent is of a similar social class and educational background to the practitioner, although the practitioner may still be inclined to use technical jargon that is not part of the educational experience of the respondent. When the respondent has limited education, or perhaps is

Box 4.3

Doctor: 'OK, so can you just run past me what you understand about what to do next?'
Patient: ' Yes, I'm going to take this form to the nurse in Casualty, and she is going to direct me to X-ray, and the doctor there is going to tell me what to do.'
Doctor: 'Yes, but after the X-ray, you need to bring the films back here for me to have a look at them. The X-ray doctor won't necessarily know that ...'

from a non-English-speaking background, the practitioner needs to use simpler words and forms of speech. It is not straightforward for a highly trained professional to use lay terms in all cases, and respondents will not necessarily indicate that they do not understand, for fear of seeming stupid. In the Consumers' Health Forum study respondents identified the use of 'plain English words that people can understand' as among the high priority, high frequency cluster of desirable attributes.[13]

A simple way to overcome difficulties related to language is to use questioning to check that everything has been understood. If it can be done easily, it is helpful to ask the listener to tell you what he or she has understood, as in Box 4.3.

This theme of checking mutual understanding is followed further in Chapter 8, Summaries and decisions.

Physical setting

The placement of the desk and chair in an interview may either impede or facilitate the flow of communication. Ideally, questioner and respondent should not be separated by a desk, or other barrier. Similarly, other features of the physical surroundings, such as lighting, the placement of a computer, and the presence of noisy interruptions may affect the interaction. In general, questioning will proceed more smoothly and freely if privacy can be assured, which is often not the case in hospital settings.

Time

Time management is vital to a good interview. Unfortunately, many interviews must be terminated before all issues are explored. Practitioners should learn a variety of ways of closing an interview, so that they do not run overtime, while structuring their questioning in such a way as to enable the patient to feel listened to and at ease.

RESPONDING TO QUESTIONS FROM THE PATIENT/CLIENT

No review of questioning in the clinical setting would be complete without a consideration of questioning from the client/patient. That such questions can and should exist need not be debated in an era where the rights of consumers have become well established. However, their role has not been fully explored. Questions by patients may vary from a simple information-seeking exercise to an attempt to share the power and decision-making in a consultation.

David Silverman conducted extensive research on patient encounters in British hospital clinics in the period 1976 to 1985. This research included a sociological analysis of the organisation of pediatric clinics and of the medical decision-making that took place in them. As part of this, he also taped and analysed more than 1200 clinic consultations.[14] His comments on the role of patient questioning are instructive. He notes that in this setting, where parents are bringing in very sick children, their questions may be more to do with practical day-to-day matters than with participation in medical decision-making. These questions are a means by which patients may assert their right to be informed. He also notes that patients' questions may be answered with a lot of information that would not normally be forthcoming. Silverman suggests that this may be due to a decision rule in operation in life-threatening situations, a rule that states: 'Tell if the patient asks.'

This suggests that clinicians should be aware of their attitudes towards patients' questions, and indeed towards the consultation as a whole. If the clinician believes that the consultation should be controlled, response to questions may be brief, and style of questioning may tend to be closed and brief. On the other hand, if the clinician approaches the consultation in a way that is more patient-centred, in which power is shared between the respondent and the clinician, then questions will tend to be more open and answers will be more forthcoming. In this way questioning can both shape and express the dynamics of the consultation.

CONCLUSION

In the first part of this chapter some ways of classifying questions according to type and function were described. Some types of questions are better suited to some functions than others, and this was described with reference to the clinical interview. Woven through this discussion was another set of considerations, to do with the use of questions by the clinician or by the patient/client in the establishment of a power relationship. The form of questions and the clinician's response to them can demonstrate either a patient-centred model, in which the power in the consultation is shared, or a doctor-centred model, in which the power rests in the hands of the clinician. As demonstrated in this chapter, patient-centred questioning might answer many of the needs of the clinician, while maintaining respect and some sense of autonomy for the patient.

NOTES

1 Hargie, O., Saunders, C. and Dickson, D. *Social Skills in Interpersonal Communication.* 3rd edn, Routledge, London, 1994.
2 Hargie, Saunders, and Dickson, 1994.
3 King, G. Open and closed questions: the reference interview, *RQ—Reference and Adult Sciences Division.* 1972, 12: pp. 157–60.
4 Gorden, R. *Basic Interviewing Skills*. Peacock Publishers, Illinois, 1992.
5 Ivey, A.E. and Simek-Downing, L. *Counseling and Psychotherapy: Skills, Theories and Practice.* Prentice-Hall, Englewood Cliffs, NJ, 1980.
6 Ivey and Simek-Downing, 1980.
7 Cohen-Cole, S.A. and Bird, J. *The Medical Interview: The Three-function Approach.* Mosby Year Book, St Louis, Missouri, 1991.
8 Consumers' Health Forum. *Integrating Consumer Views About Quality in General Practice.* Australian Government Publishing Service, Canberra, 1996.
9 Hargie, Saunders and Dickson, 1994.
10 Consumers' Health Forum, 1996.
11 Ivey and Simek-Downing, 1980.
12 Loftus, E. Leading questions and the eyewitness report, *Cognitive Psychology* 1975, 7: pp. 560–72.
13 Consumers' Health Forum, 1996.
14 Silverman, D. *Communication and Medical Practice: Social Relations in the Clinic.* Sage Publications, London, 1987.

5

Strategic searching for information

Kay Tucker

When professionals need up-to-date and relevant information, they often turn to professional manuals and journals. However, with the advent of powerful **databases** searching for information has become a more straightforward and efficient procedure. The process of searching through databases, such as those available on CD-ROM or online via the World Wide Web, which provide abstracted indexes or full text of peer reviewed articles, is described. This skill is a first step in finding information. This chapter has been contributed by a librarian who has worked in different faculty areas in major tertiary libraries both in Australia and the USA. The suggested searching strategies can be applied beyond health research.

SEARCHING STRATEGY

We live in an era of information overload. New information appears in print, audiovisual and electronic media at an alarming rate. How do you find accurate, up-to-date, and complete information that fits your requirements? Professional searchers and information specialists advocate that you follow a planned search strategy and be prepared to look in a variety of sources.

In this chapter I will provide some pointers for undertaking an initial search, a general outline for a successful search strategy, and a search example. The objective of the search demonstrated in the search example is to find current material on the legal implications of telemedicine in Australia and overseas.

The basic steps in a search strategy can be readily summarised; see Box 5.1.

1. Define your topic

Whether you are researching for an assignment, project, or an issue in the workplace, you need to accurately identify your object of search. Look closely at the issues or problems involved and isolate the key concepts that express the core of the topic you are researching. Try to think of different ways of expressing each

Box 5.1: A search strategy

1. *Define* the topic you wish to research, identifying important concepts.
2. *Determine where* you will look for information and make sure you know how to use these sources effectively.
3. *Plan* the search by identifying terms and keywords for each concept. Think of alternative ways of expressing each concept.
4. *Formulate* your search request by combining keywords using **Boolean operators** (AND, OR, NOT) and other search techniques.
5. *Perform* your search and *evaluate* your results.
6. *Refine* your search based on the evaluation of your results.
7. *Repeat* the search in other sources or databases (until you have an optimal number of relevant results).

one. Problems may be quite broad, such as in the case of determining government policy on ethical issues in health, or more specific, such as finding information on a specific disease.

Look for keywords and terms using reference books, key texts, specialised dictionaries, encyclopedias, and handbooks. If you are researching a recent or popular topic, the media can also be a useful starting point. Government reports may help you to identify concepts that need researching.

2. Determine where you will look for information and find out how to use each source effectively

This is perhaps the most important step, because if you choose an inappropriate or inadequate source, your results will be poor. The type of information you need should determine where you will search for that information. For example, to find books on your topic you will need to search in a different database compared to where you would search for journal articles. I refer to databases as collections of records that describe items such as books or journal articles, and are in electronic form.

Box 5.2

Search example—Step 1 ***Define the topic***

Concept 1—telemedicine, Concept 2—legal implications.

Books are usually likely to provide a good basic overview of your topic. A subject index within a book can be an invaluable tool to finding sections relevant to your needs. Library catalogue records now make it possible to search within the table of contents of books, thereby isolating references to specific chapters. Finding a good bibliography on your topic will also help you to identify material. These can be found at the back of most books of an academic nature. Extensive bibliographies can be published as separate volumes.

Encyclopedias or handbooks provide an overview of a topic and, as such, are a useful place to begin. They can be found in the reference collection of any larger library. For example, if you are interested in management principles, you may wish to begin by consulting an encyclopedia of management to become familiar with the terms used. Or, if you are interested in medical ethics, you might consult a dictionary of philosophy to familiarise yourself with key concepts of ethics.

Library catalogues will provide you with references to books, theses, videos, journal titles, and even evaluated Internet sites on your topic. They are predominantly now on the Web and so are there to be freely searched by anyone with an Internet connection. Libraries also have access to the National Library of Australia's database, *Kinetica*, which provides records of books, journal titles, and videos held in libraries throughout Australia. You may need to ask a librarian to check this database for you.

Most catalogues use similar search mechanisms. Information about a book is structured into records with a number of **fields**. These fields consist of, among others, the author, title, description of the book, and subject headings. Subject headings are words or phrases that describe the subject of the book. Searching using subject headings makes it more likely that you will retrieve relevant records. Be aware that different databases often use different sets of subject headings, so you will need to check the index particular to the database you are using. Library catalogues use Library of Congress Subject Headings (LCSH), although medical libraries also use MeSH (Medical Subject Headings). You will often need to search using different terms, for example *Medical Policy* (LCSH) and *Health Policy* (MeSH).

Most users start a search by simple keyword.[1] I advocate the following strategy to find appropriate subject headings, which will guide you to more accurate search results: Type in a keyword that you have identified in your search preparation. The results usually provide a brief record, with a link to a more detailed record. The detailed record will list the subject headings that have been used. On the Web, these are often hyperlinked. By clicking on the link, you will be taken to a list of records for other books on the same subject.

A good up-to-date site to find Australian libraries on the Web is at http://sunsite.berkeley.edu/Libweb/aus.html. There will be a link to the catalogue from the individual library's home page. Another good site for finding an Australian library is from the National Library at http://www.nla.gov.au/apps/libraries.

Subject guides on particular topics are produced by most libraries and are now often available on the Web. For example, from the University of New South Wales Biomedical Library web site, you can access Web-based guides by topic, leading you to relevant resources. A drop-down list will identify resources for topics such as *Health Services Management*, *Public Health*, *Health Statistics*, and so forth: http://www.library.unsw.edu.au/~biomed/resguide.html.

Journal articles are often more up-to-date than books and provide a more specific focus. To find articles relevant to your topic, you will also need to look in journal indexes, which now primarily take the form of **electronic databases**.

Databases

Databases are essential in your search for quality information. You will remember from earlier in this chapter that databases are collections of records that describe items such as books or journal articles. Many are conveniently available in electronic form. These databases are the ones that are used widely, because of their accessibility, and fast search facilities.

Some characteristics of electronic databases are:

- Content: As well as journal articles, many databases also contain records for chapters in books, theses, reports, or conference proceedings. Records may be bibliographic (i.e. information describing the item such as author, title, source, abstract) or contain the full text of the article as well as bibliographic information.
- Format: Databases can be on CD-ROM, either on stand-alone PCs or on a network, however, increasingly more are becoming available on the Web, making them much more accessible.
- Availability: Quality databases are usually available commercially by subscription, requiring a username and password. If your organisation does not subscribe to them, access may be available at your state library. Other databases are freely available on the Web. Searching subscription databases is usually more reliable than using those freely available on the Web, as they use subject descriptors and are more reliable in their updating and consistency. They also tend to extend further back in coverage.

The number of databases available is enormous, with many overlapping in content, making it difficult to decide which database to choose. Factors to consider include:

- Do you require Australian or international material?
- Does the database cover your subject area? Some databases are very specific in content (e.g. *AIDSLINE*) while others are very broad (e.g. *APAIS Health*).
- Is the time period of publications you wish to search covered by the database?

- Does the topic overlap into a different subject area? For example, if searching for information on psychological issues for patients, you should search a database that concentrates on psychology, such as *PsychInfo,* as well as the more traditional medical databases, such as *MEDLINE.*

The following popular health-related subscription databases can be accessed online via the Web. This means that they are accessible remotely from where the server storing the information is located. An authorised user is able to sit at home and access international databases as easily as those that are produced locally in Australia.[2]

International databases

MEDLINE is widely recognised as the premier source for bibliographic and abstract coverage of biomedical literature. It is produced by the National Library of Medicine in the USA and covers 1966 to the present. There are many different ways to access *MEDLINE*, some are free on the Web, while others require a subscription. Most health organisations and university libraries would have a subscription. An example of a free MEDLINE web site is provided later in this chapter.

CINAHL indexes English-language journals related to nursing and allied health fields. It has a US and international focus with some Australian content. It is produced by CINAHL Information Services and covers 1982 to the present.

PsychInfo covers the professional and academic literature in psychology and related disciplines such as medicine, psychiatry, nursing, sociology, education, pharmacology, physiology, linguistics, and other related areas. *PsycInfo* provides citations and abstracts to selected articles from more than 1300 journals, books, book chapters, dissertations, and technical reports. It is produced by the American Psychological Association.

Current Contents is the research community's pre-eminent current awareness database, providing access to tables of contents and bibliographic data from current issues of more than 7000 of the world's leading scholarly research journals in the sciences, social sciences, and arts and humanities.

BIOETHICSLINE is a database that covers the ethical, legal, and public policy issues surrounding health care and biomedical research. It is produced by the Bioethics Information Retrieval Project of the Kennedy Institute of Ethics at Georgetown University.

Australian databases

Australian databases are provided by Informit Online (http://www.informit.com.au/) using WebSpirs software. At the time of writing, full-text content has just become available for certain journals in the APAIS database, with others to follow.

Australian Public Affairs Information Service (APAIS)—Health is a subset of the APAIS database, a bibliographic database that indexes articles from published material. It covers health and medicine in Australia, and in particular, the legal, social, economic, and ethical aspects of health. It is produced by the National Library of Australia and covers 1978 to the present.

Australasian Medical Index (AMI) is a bibliographic database that indexes and abstracts articles from more than 100 Australian health and medical journals not indexed in *MEDLINE*, on all aspects of health and medicine. Coverage is from 1989 to the present.

ATSIHealth is a bibliographic database that indexes published and unpublished material on Australian indigenous health. Records relate generally to Aboriginal and Torres Strait Islander health status. It is produced at the School of Health Studies, Edith Cowan University, and covers 1988 to the present.

CINCH—Health is a subset of *CINCH*, the Australian Criminology Database. Subject coverage for *CINCH—Health* includes mental health, medical and medicolegal issues, drugs and alcohol, suicide, HIV/AIDS, corrections health, euthanasia, and occupational health and safety. It is produced by the J.V. Barry Library, Australian Institute of Criminology, and covers 1968 to the present.

DRUG indexes articles from published and unpublished material on the psychosocial aspects of substance abuse. It includes political, social, economic, psychological, and legal aspects of treatment and prevention of drug abuse (legal and illicit drugs). It is produced by the Alcohol and other Drugs Council of Australia (ADCA) and covers 1987 to the present (some material dates from 1974).

Health & Society Database (H&S) is a subset of Australian Family & Society Abstracts Database (*FAMILY*), produced by the Australian Institute of Family Studies. Subject coverage includes the health and well-being of families and individuals, health policy, health services, health education and promotion, health administration, and economic issues. It covers 1980 to the present.

RURAL is made up of five separate, smaller databases: Education for Rural Medical Practice: Goals and Opportunities; Indigenous Peoples' Health: Issues and Care in Rural and Remote Areas of the world; Rural and Remote Area Nursing; Rural and Remote Health Care; and Rural and Remote Area Aged Care. It is produced by the Australian Rural Health Research Institute at Monash University.

Serials in Australian Libraries (SIAL) allows you to search by journal title to see which libraries hold a particular journal. Many libraries also have access to these journals in electronic form.

3. Plan the search

Now that you have chosen your databases, you need to think of appropriate search terms and how you will enter them. Examine closely the concepts you have identified in Step 1 and think of as many keywords as you can to describe

Box 5.3

Search example—Step 2 ***Choose the databases***

Australian databases can be searched simultaneously using Webspirs software. Below is an example of the database selection screen supplied by the vendor Informit Online using Webspirs software to search on APAIS-health, AMI, RURAL, Health & Society.

Health (Medicine)
- [x] AMI Jul 2000 (Aust. Medical Index)
- [x] APAIS-Health May 2000 (Public Affairs)
- [ ] AusportMed May 2000 (Sports Medicine)
- [ ] CINCH-Health May 2000
- [ ] DRUG Jul 2000 (Alcohol & other Drugs)
- [x] Health_and_Society May 2000
- [x] RURAL Jun 1998 (Rural Health)

these concepts. Think of the various ways of expressing the concept. Are different spellings involved, for example, behaviour and behavior? Are there any synonyms? Think about how the words relate to one another. Do they appear as a phrase or could other words appear in between? For example, *health policy,* as well as *policy of the health department*, or *government policy on health.*

4. Formulate your search request

Most databases differ in their content but use similar types of search techniques. The symbols used may vary between databases, so the online help associated with the particular database should be consulted.

Other search techniques:

- *Truncation/wildcards*—by substituting a symbol for a number of characters in a word, the database retrieves variations of the word. This symbol is often an asterisk (*), but may be a question mark (?) or dollar sign ($). The help screens or search tips of the particular database will indicate the usage of

Box 5.4

Search example—Step 3 ***Plan the search***

Concept 1 keywords—telemedicine, telehealth, telepsychiatry
Concept 2 keywords—legal, law, laws, legislation

Box 5.5: Boolean operators

The most essential tools are *Boolean operators,* also called logical operators. These are:

- AND—finds both words in the same document or record, e.g. *telemedicine AND policy* will find records containing both the word *telemedicine* and the word *policy* anywhere in the record. Adding additional terms using AND can be useful for narrowing a search down if too many hits are retrieved.
- OR—finds either term or both terms in the document or record, e.g. *telemedicine OR telehealth* will find records with telemedicine only, *telehealth* only or both terms in the same record. Adding additional terms with OR can be useful for broadening a search or taking synonyms into account.
- NOT—finds one term but not the other term in the record, e.g. *telemedicine NOT telepsychiatry* will find records with the term *telemedicine* but not the term *telepsychiatry*. Using NOT can be useful for limiting a search to a specific area of interest.

symbols. For example *communicat** retrieves *communicate, communicates, communication, communicating,* and so forth. Care should be taken not to truncate too far as irrelevant words will be retrieved. Wildcards can take care of spelling. By typing *behavio?r* you will retrieve records with both *behavior* and *behaviour*. This technique is also useful for plurals, for example, *wom?n* retrieves *woman* and *women.*

- *Field searching*—by restricting your search to a particular field, or part of a record, such as author, title, or date more relevant results can be retrieved. The subject descriptors used by the database should be checked. Most databases have an online thesaurus, which allows you to see related subject descriptors.
- *Stop words*—searches should not be in sentence form. Instead keywords with Boolean connectors should be used. For example, instead of typing *health policy in Australia*, formulate the request as *health policy AND Australia*. Words such as *a*, *the*, *in*, and so forth are usually not recognised by databases.
- *Phrase searching*—some databases recognise a phrase if the words appear next to each other, while others require the use of quotation marks (e.g. 'health policy').

Other techniques include such operators as *NEAR/n* (to find words within a certain number of words of each other) or *w/n* (within a specified number of words of each other). The help screens or search tips for each database will provide the relevant information.

This can be a one- or multi-step process. Two steps will be used here.

Box 5.6

Search example—Step 4 Formulate the search request

Key in *telemedicine, telehealth, or telepsychiatry.*

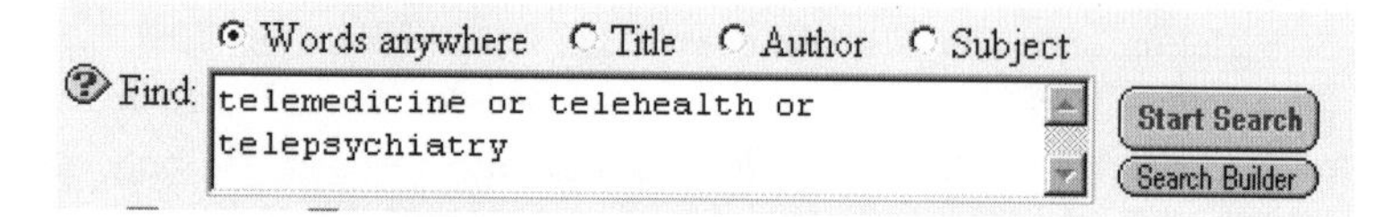

5. Perform your search and evaluate the results

Often a zero result means that you have mistyped or misspelt a word. Evaluate your results for relevance. Choose some relevant hits and look at the subject headings for further ideas on terms to use.

Box 5.7

Search example—Step 5 Perform the search and evaluate the results

Below is an example from the AMI database:

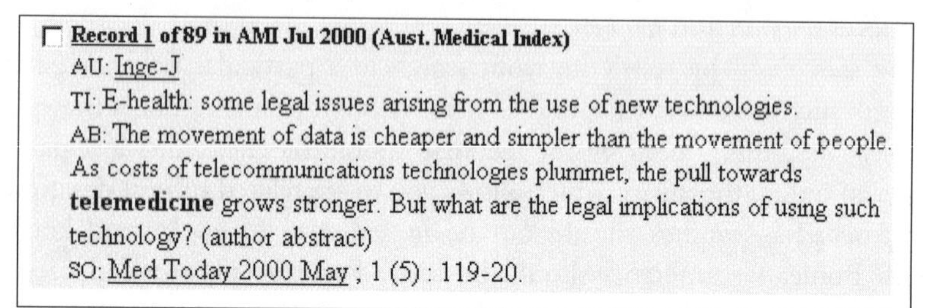

Record 1 of 89 in AMI Jul 2000 (Aust. Medical Index)

AU: Inge-J

TI: E-health: some legal issues arising from the use of new technologies.

AB: The movement of data is cheaper and simpler than the movement of people. As costs of telecommunications technologies plummet, the pull towards **telemedicine** grows stronger. But what are the legal implications of using such technology? (author abstract)

SO: Med Today 2000 May ; 1 (5) : 119-20.

Go back to the search screen and type in the keywords for Concept 2.
Key in *legal or law* or legislation.*

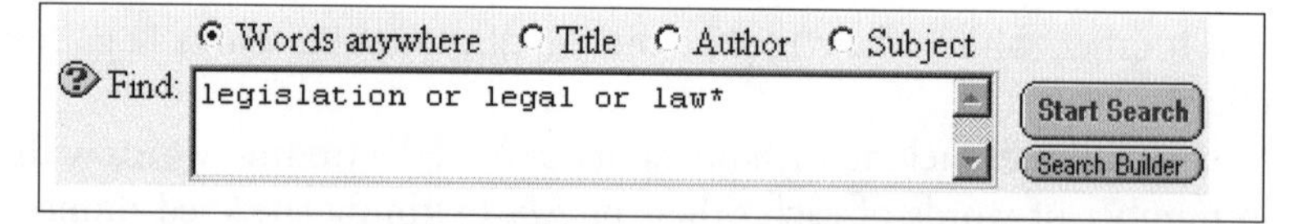

Combine the results of search #1 and search #2 to result in search #3.

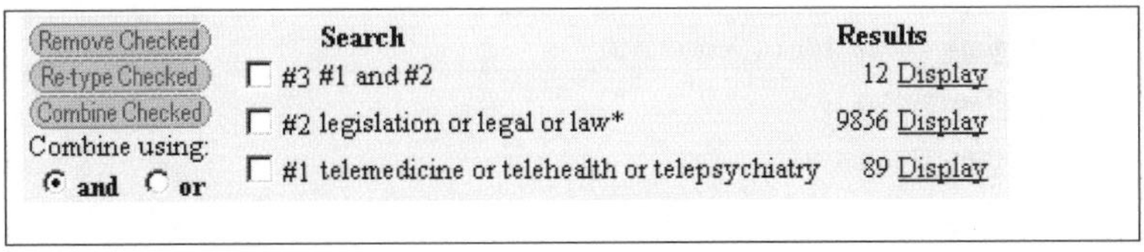

Remove Checked / Re-type Checked / Combine Checked	Search	Results
Combine using: ● and ○ or	☐ #3 #1 and #2	12 Display
	☐ #2 legislation or legal or law*	9856 Display
	☐ #1 telemedicine or telehealth or telepsychiatry	89 Display

It is rare that the first search will yield the best results, so you will generally need to move on to Step 6.

6. Refine your search strategy

A common problem is a result with far too many hits. Although the number of hits is largely dependent upon the scope of the topic and the size of the project, you should be able to restrict the search results to no more than fifty. This may mean that you need to narrow down the topic by using different terms or by adding search terms to restrict the focus of the search. Searching a particular geographic region or timespan may be helpful. On the other hand, if you are not finding enough relevant results, it may be that the database in use is not the best database for your query. A search may be broadened by considering the subject headings and choosing related areas of interest.

Box 5.8

Search example—Step 6 Refine your search if necessary

Based on your results, you may wish to add in the term *e-health* or even expand the search to *health and technology*. For legal aspects, you may also wish to search on the term *medico-legal*.

7. Repeat your search in other databases

Many people assume that they can search just one database and come up with the best results. This is by no means true. Different databases generally index different sources, although there may be some overlap. The golden rule is to try a number of databases.

Box 5.9

Search example—Step 7 Repeat search in other databases

Here the same search is made using *MEDLINE*. This example uses OVID software.

Medline 1997 to August Week 3 2000
Medline 1993 to 1996
Medline 1987 to 1992
Medline 1975 to 1986
Medline 1966 to 1974
Medline 1966 to August Week 3 2000

Select the most recent *MEDLINE* database.
Find the used subject heading by mapping the term to the Subject Heading:

Enter **Keyword** or phrase: ☑ Map Term to Subject Heading
telemedicine
Perform Search

Resulting subject heading with the number of articles using that heading. Some narrower terms are also given:

– ☑ Telemedicine (831)
☐ Remote Consultation (441)
☐ Telepathology (96)
☐ Teleradiology (262)

Look at the subheadings for the term. Choose *Legislation & Jurisprudence*:

Subheadings for: exp Telemedicine

☐ **Include All Subheadings**
-- or choose one or more of these subheadings --

☐ /cl - Classification	☐ /mt - Methods
☐ /ec - Economics	☐ /og - Organization & Administration
☐ /hi - History	☐ /st - Standards
☐ /is - Instrumentation	☐ /sn - Statistics & Numerical Data
☐ /lj - Legislation & Jurisprudence	☐ /td - Trends
☐ /ma - Manpower	☐ /ut - Utilization

Perform the search.

#	Search History	Results	Display
1	exp Telemedicine/lj [Legislation & Jurisprudence]	95	Display

Box 5.10

A subject gateway for Medicine is OMNI from the UK (http://www.omni.ac.uk). The National Library of Medicine (NLM) provides free access to more than 11 million citations in *MEDLINE* and other related databases with links to online journals. This service is called *PubMed* (http://www.ncbi.nlm.nih.gov/pubmed). From the *OMNI* site, access is available to *Pubmed* and other free Web databases as shown in the screen below:

Free MEDLINE requiring no registration

Name	Span	AT	Features	Related services	Rev
HealthGate	1966-	11s	Good variety of options on advanced search page	Several more subject-specific medical databases, some requiring registration	Yes
Infotrieve	1966-	4s	Variety of options and filters	TOXLINE, AIDSLINE, CANCERLIT	No
Internet Grateful Medline	1966-	15s	Wide variety of options. Substantial supporting documentation	Extensive collection of other medical databases	No
PubMed	???	3s	Variety of options	Limited collection of other medical databases	Yes
WebMedline	???	7s	Limited options	None	No
Snooz	???	18s	Many options; complex Java based interface	Several other databases	No

THE INTERNET

A discussion of where to find information would not be complete without mentioning the Internet. A *subject directory* should be used to facilitate your search. (Someone else has already done the searching and evaluating.) General directories such as Yahoo (http://dir.yahoo.com/Health/) provide good breakdowns by topic. *Subject gateways* are even more focused with sites selected by experts in the field.

Government sites contain a wealth of free material such as reports, fact sheets, legislation, and submissions to inquiries.

For a fairly specific topic, you may wish to use a search engine to search the Web. A university library's web site will usually provide a page with links to various search engines. Some of the more popular search engines are Northern Light, Alta Vista, Google and Webwombat (for Australian sites). There are many more. Each has different requirements for entering a search. The Help pages are useful in this respect. The Advanced Search option should be used if there is one. More important words should be entered first. Using a plus (+) to indicate 'and' is fairly standard in search engines.

Box 5.11

The Federal Government's Entry Point (http://fed.gov.au) has links to government departments. The site for the Australian Department of Health and Aged Care is at http://www.health.gov.au/.

Healthonline (http://www.health.gov.au/healthonline/index.htm) is the Department's special web site for the public and professionals. The Victorian Department of Health is at http://www.dhs.vic.gov.au and the Public Health Division is linked from there.

The results should be evaluated according to such factors as reliability and authority of the person or organisation hosting the site, its currency, and the stability of the site. (Will it still be there next year? Are there many links that do not go anywhere?). Reliable sites include those that have .edu (education), .org (organisation), or .gov (government), as part of the address. It is beyond the scope of this chapter to discuss the multitude of Internet sites available in the health care area.

The use of the Internet by professionals and patients is discussed further by Patricia Youngblood in the following chapter.

CONCLUSION

The variety of options may seem overwhelming at first. However, if the above strategy is followed, undertaking a search can be a fairly straightforward procedure. The use of a bibliographic management program such as *Endnote* (http://www.endnote.com/) is useful for recording sources. The search process can take a winding route with often surprising results, but the rewards can be immense.

NOTES

The author wishes to thank Martin Turnbull at the Victorian Department of Human Services, Public Health Division, for his advice.

1 Hersh, W. and Hickam, D.H. How well do physicians use electronic information retrieval systems? *Journal of the American Medical Association*, 1998, vol. 280, no. 15, pp. 1347–52.

2 You can read further about these and other databases in the following:
Hersh, W.R. *Information Retrieval: A Health Care Perspective.* New York: Springer, 1995.

Hutchinson, D. *MEDLINE for Health Professionals: How to Search PubMed on the Internet.* Sacramento, Cal.: New Wind Publishing, 1998.
Kiley, R. *Medical Information on the Internet: A Guide for Health Professionals.* 2nd edn, New York: Churchill Livingstone, 1999.
Ryer, J.C. *HealthNet: Your Essential Resource for the Most Up-to-date Medical Information Online.* New York: Wiley, 1997.
Wood, S.M. (ed.), *Health Care Resources on the Internet: A Guide for Librarians and Health Care Consumers.* New York: Haworth Information Press, 1999.

6

New technologies

Patricia Youngblood

We are in the age of information technology and multimedia. Communication resources have emerged that make use of these new technologies. Some of these resources are information collection points, some are support for the professional who wishes to present information or ideas in a formal setting, and some are simple communication tools that put practitioners and patients in touch with others at a distance.

Communication between patients and health care professionals is changing rapidly as new developments in computing and telecommunications technologies expand the range of possibilities for interacting in real time as well as asynchronously. In addition to improving doctors' access to the latest medical knowledge, the new technologies make it possible for doctors to conduct consultations with patients in remote areas, to monitor chronically ill patients in their homes, and to encourage patients to become more informed in ways of preventing illness and promoting good health.

NEW COMMUNICATION TECHNOLOGIES

In the past, health professionals have relied predominantly on the telephone and postal service, colloquially called 'snail mail', to deliver their messages to patients and colleagues. With the advent of new communication technologies, the options have expanded dramatically. It is now possible to communicate in real time with one or more persons simultaneously via audio teleconferencing, videoconferencing, computer conferencing or in online chat rooms. It is also possible to enrich these interactions with a full range of media, including high-resolution visual images, digitised audio, and full motion video. Alternatively, we can send messages to be received at a later time using voicemail, facsimile, **electronic mail** (email), bulletin boards, or online discussion groups. As these options expand, we must learn more about each mode of communication, so we can choose the best medium for our communication needs.

Table 6.1: Synchronous and asynchronous communication[1]

	Sound	*Image*	*Data*
Synchronous	telephony	video-conferencing	shared electronic whiteboards, shared documents
Asynchronous	voicemail	letter and notes, computer image store and forward	paging, fax, email

We might begin thinking about communication needs by looking at where and when the communication takes place. These interactions are often classified into 'synchronous' and 'asynchronous' events (see Table 6.1). **Synchronous communication** occurs when the individuals communicate in real time, as in a face-to-face or phone conversation. **Asynchronous communication** occurs when individuals are separated by time and/or distance, as in written or voice-mail messages.

SYNCHRONOUS COMMUNICATION

We know that the most effective communication between individuals occurs when there is a two-way interaction. When this happens, there are many opportunities to talk, to listen, and to ask questions. It follows that synchronous or real-time communication is often preferred, especially in the case of health professionals consulting with their clients and colleagues. **Telephony** is the term used to describe the use of telephone lines for two-way communication between individuals who are separated by distance, but wish to communicate in real time. While the telephone has been with us for quite some time now, new developments in mobile telephony make it possible not only to reach people more easily, but also to access data via the **Internet** and the **World Wide Web** using wireless channels.[2]

Teleconferencing, videoconferencing, and healthcare

Synchronous communication among health professionals was previously limited to office consultations and telephone conversations. However, advances in teleconferencing technologies now allow us to expand this option to include communication among groups of people who are geographically dispersed, and the ability to incorporate a variety of media, or multimedia, in these interactions.

The use of communication technologies in health care is referred to as '**telemedicine**' or sometimes 'telehealth'. As Coiera explains, *'The essence of* *telemedicine is the exchange of information at a distance, whether that information is voice, an image, elements of a medical record, or command to a surgical robot. It seems reasonable to think of telemedicine as the remote communication of information to facilitate clinical care.'*[3] Although initially criticised as being too expensive to be practical, telemedicine and telehealth are certain to be expanding areas in the twenty-first century. This technology has already proved to be especially useful in large countries with a dispersed population, such as Australia and Canada, where there are remote regions with limited access to health care resources, especially medical specialists.

There are now applications in many fields of health, especially where the transmission of visual media is important. These include teleradiology, teledermatology, telepathology, and teleophthalmology.[4] According to Angaran, telepharmacy is also a growth area and refers to the use of electronic information and communications technologies to support pharmaceutical care provision. He explains that while videoconferencing is being used for education, training, and management purposes, the telephone has become a multimedia access tool. *'Medical devices are being attached to telephone lines to provide remote monitoring and therapy, and call centers are providing medication counseling, prior authorization, refill authorization, and formulary compliance monitoring.'*[5]

Coiera provides a more detailed description of this significant development in the application of telecommunication technology in health care—remote monitoring of patients in their homes.[6] These services range from a regularly scheduled phone call to check on patients recently released from hospital, to the use of automatic voicemail reminders to help elderly patients remember to take their medications. More complex monitoring systems are also being developed, including monitoring equipment installed in the home that takes measurements such as blood pressure and cardiogram data and transmits the data to remote monitoring stations.[7] These services make it possible for patients who have suffered an acute episode such as an **infarction** (e.g. a heart attack or stroke) to be discharged from hospital earlier and for elderly or chronically ill patients to be managed effectively in their homes.

Shared documents and shared electronic whiteboards

In the same way that videoconferencing expands upon teleconferencing by adding visual images, shared documents and shared electronic whiteboards provide two or more individuals with synchronous access to the same data and the same workspace. These technologies enrich the nature of the remote clinical consultation by allowing the individuals to write or draw on a shared visual screen and to access laboratory data and other results that have been stored in electronic format. As seen in industry, the ability to share documents and work space is also extremely useful in project management and problem-solving, for example among health professionals who are geographically dispersed.

ASYNCHRONOUS COMMUNICATION

The technologies that support communication across time and distance include voicemail, electronic mail, mailing lists, newsgroups, and bulletin boards. Perhaps the most significant of these is the rapid expansion in the use of electronic mail, usually termed 'email', by health professionals and the public in general. A recent survey of online health information users in the USA revealed that 50 per cent of users would like to be able to access a doctor's web site and 48 per cent said they would like to be able to email their doctor's office (http://www.cyberdialogue.com).

However, doctors remain cautious about the potential legal and ethical implications of using the Internet to communicate with patients. Spielberg warns that physicians using email should be aware of '*the new expectations, practice standards, and potential liabilities that emerge with the introduction of this new communication technology*'.[8] She notes especially that email communications may be included in the patient's medical record, and recommends that physicians gain informed consent before using email. In addition they must take precautions to maintain the confidentiality of patient information that is shared in this form of communication.

Some additional ways in which the Internet is being used for asynchronous communication between groups of people include mailing lists, newsgroups, and bulletin boards. Mailing lists can be used to participate in an online group discussion. Any individual in the group may send an email message to the moderator for distribution to the other members of the group. The moderator is then responsible for reviewing all messages for appropriateness before distributing the messages to the other group members, and for maintaining the list of group members.[9]

Newsgroups and bulletin boards provide another way for groups of individuals to communicate online. As with mailing lists, a moderator reviews messages that are posted to the group and maintains the list of 'subscribers' to these groups. However, instead of being mailed to each of the group members, the electronic messages are posted to the newsgroup or bulletin board, which is a central location on the network. In this way, anyone who has subscribed to the group will be able to read all messages posted, as well as send messages to be reviewed and posted.[10]

Gilas et al. conducted a retrospective review of an Internet discussion list for surgeons, called Surginet. In 1997 Surginet was the largest medical discussion list on the Internet dealing with general surgery. At that time it had 489 subscribers from 46 countries. The authors distributed a questionnaire to all subscribers to determine their perceptions of the usefulness of this form of communication among health professionals. Their conclusions are as follows:

> Groups such as Surginet fill a niche involving free exchange of ideas, methods, and attitudes relevant to the current practice of general surgery, which is different from the way medical information is disseminated by published literature and organised medical meetings. There is a perception among list subscribers that this is a valuable and useful modality for continuing education.[11]

IMPLICATIONS FOR PATIENTS

Greater access to health information

As health care issues become increasingly complex, patients are becoming more interested in learning about their conditions and illnesses so they can make wise choices about treatment options. The Internet and World Wide Web make it easier for patients and their carers to access health information from an ever-increasing number of health care web sites in Australia and around the world. Health insurance providers are also supporting this move towards increased patient education and patient empowerment in managing their own health.

A 1999 survey of Internet users in the USA showed that 33 per cent of all US adults are online and that 38 per cent of this group have used the Internet for health and medical information over the last twelve months (http://www.cyber-dialogue.com). In 1995, 3.2 million adults in the USA used the Internet for health and medical information, rising to 24.8 million adults in 1999. This increase has been used to project an estimate of 52.0 million adult 'health users' by 2003. The survey documents the trend among consumers, particularly those younger than 50 years of age, to take a greater role in the management of their health.[12]

The Internet seems to be both a catalyst and a symptom of a change in consumer attitudes about their doctors. Those who use the Internet for health information are more likely to express the attitude that '*the patient needs to take primary responsibility for his or her health and not rely as much on doctors*'.[13] This attitude is reflected in the increasing number of patients who bring Internet health information with them to discuss during their doctor visits, especially in the area of pharmaceuticals.

Finally, the survey showed that Internet health consumers '*would most like to retrieve their online health information from their doctors, ahead of national medical center experts, insurance companies, drug companies and new Internet companies (all of whom are currently providing much of the health information online).*'[14]

Surfing the net?

Low back pain

www.jr2.ox.ac.uk?Bandolier/band19/b19-1.html

Low back pain, general interest sponsored by the University of Oxford

www.spine-surgery.com

On line discussion group sponsored by Spine Surgery, Louisville Kentucky

www.vh.radiology.uiowa.edu

patient education materials on back pain management; useful links to other sites sponsored by the University of Iowa College of Medicine

www.srs.org

Scoliosis (spinal deformity)

Figure 6.1 Web site addresses for low back pain management

Source: Office of Michael Ryan, MS, FRACS, Orthopaedic Surgeon, North Shore Medical Centre, 66 Pacific Highway, St. Leonards, NSW, 2065.

One easy way to respond to consumer needs in this area is for health care providers to recommend appropriate web sites to their patients. On a recent visit to an orthopaedic surgeon's office in Sydney, I found a list of web sites for patients suffering from low back pain. The list, which was prepared by the doctor himself, is reproduced in Figure 6.1.

Online patient support groups

As shown above, many comprehensive health information web sites offer not only information about illness and disease, but also a way of contacting others with similar problems for support and advice. These online patient support groups have enormous potential for helping improve patients' quality of life.

A recent research study at the Patient Education Research Center at Stanford University is exploring the ways in which an online patient support group for people with chronic low back pain may have an impact on health outcomes including a reduction in health care utilisation. This randomised two-year study consists of an email news group that includes a physician, physiotherapist, and psychologist, as well as two moderators as members of the group. The group participants discuss any issues they have related to back pain. The health professionals comment but will not give specific medical advice. Those accepted into the study include people who suffer from recurrent back pain, but have not had any surgical treatment for their problem. The researchers will follow these individuals for a three-year period, recording information about their health behaviours, health status, health care utilisation, and days lost from work. Kate Lorig is the principal investigator and Diana Laurent is the study coordinator.[15] (For more information, see the Stanford Center's web site—http://www.stanford.edu/ group/perc/).

A program in the United Kingdom called DIPEx demonstrates yet another variation on the use of new technologies to inform and support patients.[16] The authors describe the intervention as follows:

> The Database of Individual Patients' Experience of illness (DIPEx) is a multimedia web site and CD-ROM that links patients' experiences with evidence-based information about treatments and the illness itself and with a range of other resources that may be useful, including support groups and links to other web sites. DIPEx aims to identify the questions that matter to people when they are ill and it has the potential for informing patients, educating healthcare professionals, and providing a patient-centred perspective to researchers and those who manage health services.[17]

A WORD OF CAUTION

While the potential of the new technologies for promoting health and preventing disease is great, there are some important obstacles that will need to be addressed. Eng et al. point out, for example that those members of the community who have preventable health problems and have no health insurance coverage are the least likely group to have access to these technologies. They suggest that barriers to accessing online health information include *'cost, geographic location, illiteracy, disability, and factors related to the capacity of people to use these technologies appropriately and effectively'.*[18]

Jadad and Gagliardi suggest that despite the benefits, the availability of health information on the Internet carries the potential for harmful effects on both consumers and health professionals.[19] Their concern is with the quality of incompletely developed instruments to evaluate health information on the Internet. Their analysis of forty-seven rating instruments showed that only fourteen provided a description of the criteria used to produce the ratings and none provided information on **interobserver reliability** and **construct validity** of the measurements.

Winker et al. share this concern for the accuracy of information provided via the Internet.[20] They acknowledge the impact of better access to health information on the changing nature of the doctor–patient relationship, including a trend towards shared decision-making. However, barriers impeding progress in this area include:

> wide variations in quality of content on the Web, potential for commercial interests to influence online content, and uncertain preservation of personal privacy. To address these issues, the American Medical Association has developed principles to guide the development and posting of Web site content, govern acquisition and posting of online advertising and sponsorship, ensure site visitors' and

patients' rights to privacy and confidentiality, and provide effective and secure means of e-commerce.[21]

INTERACTION CHANGES

As more and more people become computer literate and gain access to the ever increasing amount of health information available on the World Wide Web, they are becoming more informed and therefore more empowered to become active partners with their health professionals in the management of their health. This shift in the relationship between patients and their health care providers necessitates a change in communication patterns, where the opportunity to share information and discuss options becomes increasingly important.

The consultation between patient and provider in the future is likely to include a review of health web sites and other relevant online information resources.

NOTES

1 Reproduced from E. Coiera, 1997, *Guide to Medical Informatics, the Internet and Telemedicine*. Arnold Publishers, London, p. 199.
2 Coiera, E. 1997, p. 216.
3 Coiera, E. 1997, p. 224.
4 Stanberry, B. 2000. Telemedicine: barriers and opportunities in the 21st century. *Journal of Internal Medicine,* 247 (6): pp. 615–28.
5 Angaran, D. 1999. Telemedicine and telepharmacy: current status and future implications. *American Journal of Health–System Pharmacy,* 56 (14) pp. 1405–26, p. 1405.
6 Coiera, E. 1997, pp. 227–8.
7 Rodriquez, M.J., Martinz, A. and Dopico, A. 1995. A home telecare management system, Doughty, K., Cameron, K. Gardner P. 1996 Three generations of telecare of the elderly, *Journal of Telemedicine & Telecare* 2(2) pp. 71–80 in Coiera, 1997, p. 228.
8 Spielberg, A. 1998. On call and online: sociohistorical, legal and ethical implications of email for the patient–physician relationship, *Journal of the American Medical Association,* 280 (15): pp. 1353–9.
9 Coiera, E. 1997, pp. 253–4.
10 Coiera, E. 1997, pp. 254–5.
11 Gilas, T., Schein, M. and Frykberg, E. 1998. A surgical Internet discussion list (Surginet): a novel venue for international communication among surgeons. *Archives of Surgery,* 133 (10): pp. 1126–30.
12 Reents, S. (1999) *Impacts of the Internet on the Doctor–Patient Relationship: The Rise of the Internet Health Consumer* (http://www.cyberdialogue.com).

13 Ibid., p.3.
14 Ibid., p. 5.
15 Lorig, K., August 29, 2000. Personal email communication. Further information available from the Stanford Patient Education Research Center, Stanford University: http://www.stanford.edu/group/perc/perchome.html
16 Herxheimer, A., McPherson, A., Miller, R., Shepperd, S., Yaphe, J. and Ziebland, S. 2000. Database of patients' experiences (DIPEx): a multi-media approach to sharing experiences and information, *The Lancet* 355(9214): pp. 1540–43.
17 Herxheimer A. et al. 2000, p. 1540.
18 Eng, T., Maxfield, A., Patrick, K., Deering, M., Ratzan, S. and Gustafson, D. 1998. Access to health information and support: a public highway or private road? *Journal of the American Medical Association*, 280 (15): 1371–5, p. 1371.
19 Jadad, A., Gagliardi, A. 1998. Rating health information on the Internet: navigating to knowledge or to Babel? *Journal of the American Medical Association*, 279 (8): pp. 611–14.
20 Winker, M., Flanagin, A., Chi-Lum, B., White, J., Andrews, K., Kennett, R., DeAngelis, C. and Musacchio, R. 2000. Guidelines for medical and health information sites on the Internet: principles governing AMA web sites, *Journal of the American Medical Association,* 283 (12): pp. 1600–6.
21 Winker, M., et al. 2000, p. 1600.

7

Analysis—making sense of what happens

Peter Harris

The task of analysing is a responsibility of all health care professionals. Gathering information is one step. Interpreting and rechecking the information is also crucial. This draws on the professional expertise, and communication skill, of the practitioner. Relevant information can only be gathered with appropriate knowledge backing that process. Checking the accuracy and relevance of information needs considerable reflective ability and subtle communication skill. This chapter has been contributed by a clinical educator who is also a general practitioner. It is written with the general practice context in mind. However, the general term 'clinician' is used throughout as the principles and evidence relate across disciplines and not solely to medical consultations. The concepts are very useful for all health care professionals, and particularly for those in other ambulatory care settings.

INTERACTION

The start of most ambulatory interactions is the planned appointment. A patient comes to see a doctor with a health concern. Chapters 3 and 4 offered detailed advice on strategies to elicit the patient's initial concerns. This will not be repeated here. It is simply noted that the process of eliciting concerns takes some time.

The importance of listening and questioning skills, however, extends beyond the initial stage of a consultation. These are central communication skills because they are intertwined with the process of clinical analysis.

CONSULTATION TASKS

Once the clinician is satisfied that the patient's reason for attending has been elicited, the next phase of the interaction is to interpret these data and organise

Box 7.1

The tasks of the consultation are to:

- recognise the patient's suffering;
- conduct a diagnostic search;
- name the illness; and
- move from thinking about the cause to thinking about healing.[1]

them in a manner that is meaningful for the clinician (see Box 7.1). This is the analytic phase of the consultation. The analysis is directed towards achieving the tasks of the consultation.

As this book deals with communication in health care, it is useful to employ a task approach described by McWhinney to organise the analytic phase of the consultation. Communication occurs between people and is part of a context. The interactivity and context inform and drive the process of analysis of the clinician. It is by following the tasks that the perspectives of both patient and clinician can be brought together towards a useful outcome for the interaction.

These tasks include the usually described tasks of diagnosis and management but go beyond these more mechanistic descriptors to encompass the personal interaction included in the clinician's task. Each phase will be explored in this chapter.

The tasks are not linear despite the implications of the list above. Rather, they oscillate between listening, questioning, and analysing. The clinician will form hypotheses from the moment of first greeting the patient, if not before, and will be testing these hypotheses while inviting the patient to tell his or her story. Elements such as gait, demeanour, facial expression, and punctuality all form patterns for the experienced clinician, even before a word is exchanged. Consultations during a particular season or during an epidemic also create hypotheses in the mind of the clinician of what the health issue may be for each patient.

Such hypotheses are tested, and new ones formulated, as the patient's story unfolds, without the clinician necessarily asking any questions at this time. This testing continues throughout the interchange, and during the clinical examination. The **hypothesis** testing continues after the physical consultation has been concluded, when test results are analysed or at follow-up visits. The questioning becomes more focused as analyses are interpreted to form a pattern and new data reinforce the pattern or challenge its validity, which in turn triggers more listening.

A historical shift

The tasks of the consultation have been described over the last half century as 'diagnosis, diagnosis, diagnosis'.[2] Thinking about the role of the clinician in this interaction has been as influential in broadening this approach as technology has been in transforming the diagnostic task itself.[3] While patients have been at the centre of the consultation, a narrower method expressed as 'find it and fix it' resulted from effective medical therapies and safe surgery.[4] Clinicians in the latter part of the twentieth century have been more clearly focused onto what has come to be called a **patient-centred clinical method** and have developed a language to express this method.

RECOGNISING THE PATIENT'S SUFFERING

An understanding of the patient and his or her situation is central to the communication between clinician and patient. Patients come to a consultation with their own understandings and beliefs about their situation. They have usually gone through their own process of analysis. This often includes seeking other advice about their situation, usually from family members or trusted friends.[5]

Patients bring a set of questions to the interaction that are different from those that the clinician usually asks. Box 7.2 sets out some examples of questions that may be in the mind of the patient or the clinician. Notice that they may be unspoken.

Schumacher contends that people who have never consciously experienced a condition could not possibly know about another person's experience of the condition.[6] The outward signs would be noted, but they would be unable to understand them correctly independently. They would attempt some kind of interpretation that may or may not reflect the reality of the patient.

Box 7.2

Examples of questions

In a patient's mind
- What is happening to me?
- Why is this happening?
- Will I be able to continue my activities?
- Will this affect my family?

In a clinician's mind
- What is the diagnosis?
- What are the risk factors?
- What is the treatment?

Empathy is probably the next best thing. The most frequently expressed cause for satisfaction of a consultation is a sense of being listened to, or, even better, understood. While understanding is not always possible, the art of listening contributes profoundly to the consultation. This becomes the first point of 'diagnosis' in most consultations, that of developing an understanding of the patient. Without this sense of the patient as a person, the later understanding of the condition is less efficient, or is less likely to be correct.

One of the tasks undertaken by clinicians, which has been identified by studying clinicians' interactions with patients, is that of 'interactive reasoning'. This is the task of seeking to understand the patient as an individual, and seeking to understand the meaning of the illness for that person. This interactive process is often more intuitive than a recognisable part of an analysis. For this reason it is less likely to be discussed as part of the interaction and may not even be recognised by the clinician. If the clinician is focused on the 'best treatment', this interactive engagement of the patient may not be acknowledged. This task may be conducted subconsciously. Many elements of the interaction provide data that are processed leading towards an individualised outcome (or plan) for the consultation.

The language of the patient opens a window to their experience for the clinician to observe and, where appropriate, interpret. This glimpse will not usually yield understanding but allows contact with the experience from the patient's perspective. Language, both verbal and non-verbal, reveals the extent and depth of a symptom, its impact on the patient's life and psyche as well as the physical effect. For example, the clenched fist on the chest reveals more about the nature of chest pain than a five-minute description employing all the published metaphors. The anxiety in the patient's tone encourages the first clinical interpretation of 'is this urgent?'

More usually, the language used to express a problem holds clues to the patient's understanding of the problem, its seriousness, or its cause. The term 'a touch of sugar' reveals much of that patient's attitude to diabetes and may point to their belief about management and adherence to a dietary regime. Here the clinician's use of reflection and exploratory open questioning should reveal enough to determine the direction of the next phase of this consultation. At this point the patient should be encouraged to feel comfortable and allowed sufficient time to describe their beliefs and expectations about their situation.

Patients' beliefs impact on their likelihood to follow a particular path of management, or even to accept a particular diagnostic label. These are discussed in more detail below and again highlight the non-linear nature of clinical interpretation. Indeed, informed consent is not possible if the patient and the clinician do not share an understanding of the nature of the condition that they are dealing with.

CONDUCTING A DIAGNOSTIC SEARCH

The scan and search strategy of the opening phase of the clinician's activity relies on a variety of formulated hypotheses. Efficient interaction allows the patient to explain their presentation and condition, before interruption by the clinician.[7] Initial patient descriptions are accompanied by the clinician's silent searching for signs of urgency, danger, and probability. All too frequently the literature informs us that the clinician does not wait for these signs to form, but interrupts the opening patient narrative to meet their own agenda. This searching process includes more than just gathering information that could be obtained from a letter or telephone call.

The tasks may differ somewhat according to the role of the clinician. A general practitioner will explore probability and marginalise danger; a specialist seeing a referred patient will seek to explore possibility and marginalise error.[8] The generalist tolerates uncertainty and has high **sensitivity**, while the specialist reduces uncertainty to increase **specificity**.

While using the scan and search method, the clinician has multiple hypotheses and applies a probabilistic evaluation of the emerging data. These data are tested against a range of hypotheses, almost simultaneously, to lend weight to one and reduce the likelihood of another. Here also the process interacts with the dynamic between clinician and patient. Throughout the ebb and flow of problem-solving, classifications that the clinician recognises and finds useful are gradually formed. Classifications with minimal probability of being useful are sifted for rejection.

The hypotheses that are being tested are not just those of the underlying pathology. The exploration is broader than a physical, or technical, concern.

Box 7.3

What is routinely being explored?

- the pathological state
- the patient's reaction to that state
- the patient's readiness to be active in altering their situation

What provides clues?

- careful observation of the patient
- the patient's explanation of their predicament
- the words and body language employed
- the manner and cadence of the presentation

Each activity or exploration requires a different level of observation and processing. These are not usually described as analysis, but contribute to the clinician's understanding of the patient and their problem, so in reality are the analysis.

Initial scanning and classification usually starts with an urgent or non-urgent binary choice. Like many choices that follow, the classification reflects some proposed or potential action rather than a neat systematic or hierarchical structure. For example, the central decision in upper respiratory infection can be viewed as a decision to prescribe medication, or not to prescribe.[9] If this is accepted as the ultimate decision structure by the clinician, then it is likely that the other clinical details available in a consultation are shaped around this action-oriented choice.

In practice, then, the process of diagnostic search is about testing a series of preliminary decisions, or best fit. Much of the action that follows in the next phase will be decided by a series of binary choices.

NAMING THE ILLNESS

The 'naming the illness' phase of the analysis most closely corresponds to the 'diagnosis' of traditional teaching. It is generally accepted that an accurate diagnosis is the beginning of effective treatment. It is also generally accepted that knowing what the problem is allows the application of tested remedies. These assumptions should be subjected to critical analysis (see Box 7.4).

Box 7.4

These statements are correct when:

- we can be sure that the diagnosis represents the clinical situation of the patient; and
- there are tried and effective remedies; and
- the remedies fit the patient.

The diagnosis is useful for us to compare similar diseases, to gather information about prognosis, and to employ effective treatments. The strength of a diagnosis lies in its predictive power. An understanding of organic pathology and skilful use of laboratory tests and imaging increase our ability to identify conditions accurately.

Patients seek to understand what is happening to them and usually desire some explanation. Such explanation is usually preceded by giving the patient's distress a name. The process of naming can have both positive and negative effects on the outcome. Patients seek an explanation and both patient and clinician may be comforted by a diagnostic label. This may be so even if the label is no more than a description of the symptoms, as in for instance, irritable bowel syndrome, or sciatica. They can share the delusion that they understand and have therefore controlled the predicament of that patient's presentation.

Conversely, Sackett and Haynes describe adverse outcomes from identification and naming in children with heart murmurs. Those children who were later found to have no pathology had as much disability in terms of their activity as those children who were later confirmed to have cardiac disease.[10]

This is the paradox of the 'diagnosis'. Organic pathology and diagnosis are related, yet the patient has an experience different from that of another person with the same organic pathology.

From a mechanistic view, a lack of agreement on the problem hinders management. The person with asthma, who denies their diagnosis, will continue to cough and wheeze, even when they obtain antibiotics for their 'bronchitis'. At a deeper level, the patient is trying to make sense of this episode in their world. The clinician needs to find a way to access the patient's understanding and beliefs. The patient with a family history of thyroid cancer who is told that their neck lumps are benign lymphadenopathy will remain as concerned, and may resent what they see as lack of concern or clinical skill.

The skilled clinician moves rapidly from the exposition of diagnosis to its impact on the patient. Statements such as 'You seem concerned. Are you wondering if this is something serious?' provide opportunities for patients to expose and explore their concerns and arrive at a common understanding with their clinicians about the nature of their problem.

Clinicians are frequently reported to appear to jump from the physical to the interpersonal to the context. This phenomenon has been described in occupational therapy where there seem to be (at least) three 'different tracks' operating simultaneously.[11] The skilful clinician moves from one track to another in response to signals from the patient. The clinician is then able to resume their pursuit of the previous agenda when the patient's new issues are dealt with.

This agility is not random as it may appear to a casual observer. It is a blend of awareness of the patient, the pathologic probabilities, and the context of the illness. The tracks may not all operate consciously at once and probably do not employ the same analytical skills used to test diagnostic hypotheses.

The nature of the clinical setting is that hypotheses are entertained in multiples. Elstein et al. identified that clinicians use four important features to solve diagnostic problems.[12] These are cue identification, hypothesis generation, cue interpretation, and hypothesis evaluation. Of these four, the only constant feature was the use of multiple hypotheses. These competing formulations (differential diagnosis or alternative diagnoses) are tested against each other by seeking further cues especially by use of refuting questions.[13] The refuting question asks about a feature that could not be present if the diagnosis in question is accurate. As there are relatively few accurate refuting questions, clinicians routinely seek the presence or absence of positive features of the diagnosis. Questions that discriminate between diagnoses are an efficient strategy for sorting predetermined categories. They do not deal with other possibilities that were not entertained as part of the differential diagnosis.

For the multiple competing hypotheses to be efficient, clinicians move through a series of 'problem spaces',[14] with larger spaces being either organ systems (e.g. cardiovascular system), symptom clusters (e.g. shortness of breath), or regional anatomy (e.g. the abdomen). They rapidly move into smaller and smaller spaces by testing the competing hypotheses. The more expert the clinician, the more cues are recognised early and the less reliance is placed on inference, with a greater bank of patterns being employed as the test of competing hypotheses.

In a significant number of general-practice consultations, and in many consultations with allied health professionals, a traditional 'diagnosis' is not named. This may be because the presentation is an early undifferentiated condition still evolving, a brief self-limiting condition, or an exacerbation of an ongoing condition where the original diagnosis is largely irrelevant. It may be that the problem presented is not in the 'find it and fix it' paradigm. Rather, the clinician and the patient arrive at a common understanding of the nature of the patient's predicament by iterative discussion about this predicament and its implications. From there they can move to responding to this predicament in some way.

The skilful clinician incorporates ongoing questioning or scepticism about the diagnostic hypotheses, especially as a diagnosis is approaching. Significant errors can result from the initial assumptions on which the searching is based. A patient with abdominal pain during a gastroenteritis epidemic may still have appendicitis. An incorrect early assumption about the context of the presentation may result in a serious misdiagnosis.

The process of forming a therapeutic alliance between the clinician and the patient begins with the clinician describing their understanding of the problem, their plans for the next step(s) and a division of labour setting out roles for this management.

MOVING FROM THINKING ABOUT THE CAUSE TO THINKING ABOUT HEALING

Consultations conclude with a management plan, not with a diagnosis. Whether or not there is a therapeutic intervention, both clinician and patient need to understand the plan of action after the consultation. If a diagnosis has been made, the clinician is able to provide some estimate of the likely course of this predicament and identify any appropriate interventions. At this stage in a consultation it is usual for the clinician to have more 'air time' than the patient.

If the relationship has been well established earlier in the consultation and agreement reached on the likely nature of the predicament, then a plan can be rapidly negotiated. A provisional management plan has been in evolution from the initial description of the problem. As we have seen, early assumptions about management tend to shape the search strategies and diagnostic hypotheses. The clinician and the patient have been exchanging signals about what may be acceptable as management in this situation. The evolution of this management plan is driven by those interpersonal observations made along the way as well as by the diagnostic categories. It is a part of the iterative journey undertaken by clinician and patient.

The clinician needs to return to the reason for the consultation. Patients arrive at a consultation with symptoms and concerns and these must be dealt with during the encounter. A patient's expectations at the start of the consultation may be modified by the process of reaching a common understanding. A patient presenting with a headache, and seeking short-term analgesia, who is found to have elevated blood pressure, may be content to modify their activities and review their blood pressure at a later date. The initial request for analgesia needs to be checked again to determine if that need still exists, or if it has been satisfied by the explanation and relationship between the clinician and the patient. Patient preferences and concerns are explicitly sought and the clinician is able to express his or her own view of relative advantages and limitations of management options. Such a relationship has been described as mutuality.[15] This increases the commitment of both parties to any agreed plan.

Moving on from concern about cause to action towards healing requires a focus on the common goals and a pathway towards them. These goals may be about maintaining quality of life, or reducing exacerbations, or they may be about cure.

Cues from the patient suggest how much the patient wishes to know about the condition presented, and the extent to which participation in decision-making about management is desired. These cues deserve to be checked to avoid misinterpretation or paternalism.

The final piece of analysis in moving towards healing is checking that the patient understands the plan. In simple terms, asking about the doses and timing of medication will reveal much about the previous communication. More complex decisions need greater awareness by the clinician of vocal hesitation, body language, and those impressions of the person that do not arise from a purely 'analytical' approach to the patient, but tap into the other track of personal reaction and understanding. Here the very act of personal contact has been described as a therapeutic tool, the 'doctor as drug'.[16]

However potent the therapeutic options, it is the patient who has to heal. Healing is more than the eradication of disease. Antibiotics may remove an invading bacterium but patients vary in their recovery time and degree of disability. Management is individualised to that particular patient at that particular time with that particular problem by an understanding of the physical and social context of the patient. Patient presentations have a context. Social and psychological factors contribute to the cause of illness and can equally contribute to resolution. Careful questioning may be required to clarify these various contexts throughout the consultation.

CONCLUSION

Research into the reasoning process has often, quite understandably, focused on the task of improving clinical judgment and diagnostic accuracy by systematic analysis of the process. One consequence of this approach has been a search for 'the best strategy' for analysing patient problems and a statistical investigation of observed phenomena. While the search for improved diagnostic accuracy is important, this approach does not address the 'complexity and possibly elusive character of medical reasoning'.[17]

The idea of various parallel tracks allows one to conceptualise the leaps from biological, psychological, interpersonal, and contextual levels at which a consultation is analysed. This analysis becomes integrated in a commonly agreed plan of management for the individual. The clinician moves from one level to another in response to signals from the patient. A skilful clinician is constantly monitoring and analysing these signals using their various senses and unconscious personal responses.

Diagnostic categories are systems that belong in the world of clinicians and help them understand the biological or behavioural problem. They are not a part of the patient's world and do not explain the meaning or extent of an illness for an individual. The tasks for the clinician require movement between the clinical world-view and the patient's reality.

This interaction between clinician and patient is rich and complex. It deserves more observation and attention in an attempt to understand this richness. More 'analysis' in the traditional sense, may not provide the answers we seek.

NOTES

1 McWhinney, I. *A Textbook of Family Medicine.* New York: Oxford University Press, 1989.

2 Marinker, M. Looking and leaping, in M. Marinker and M. Peckham (eds), *Clinical Futures.* London: British Medical Association, 1998, p. 12.

3 Stewart, M., Brown, J.B., Weston, W.W., McWhinney, I.R., McWilliam, C.L. and Freeman, T.R. *Patient Centred Medicine.* Thousand Oaks, Cal.: Sage, 1995.

4 Silverman, J., Kurtz, S. and Draper, J. *Skills for Communicating with Patients.* Oxon: Radcliffe Medical Press, 1998.

5 George, J. and Davis, A. *States of Health: Health and Illness in Australia.* 3rd edn, Melbourne: Addison Wesley Longman, 1998.

6 Schumacher, E.F. *Guide to the Perplexed.* New York: Harper & Row, 1977.

7 Beckman, H.B. and Frankel, R.N. The effect of physician behaviour on the collection of data. *Annals of Internal Medicine* 1984, vol. 101, p. 692.

8 Marinker, M. Looking and Leaping, in M. Marinker and M. Peckham (eds), *Clinical Futures.* London: British Medical Association, 1998.

9 Howie, J.G. A new look at respiratory illness in general practice, *Journal of the Royal College of General Practitioners* 1973, vol. 23, p. 895.

10 Sackett, D.L. and Haynes, R.B. *Clinical Epidemiology: A Basic Science for Clinical Medicine,* Boston: Little, Brown, 1985.

11 Fleming, M.H. The therapist with the three track mind. *American Journal of Occupational Therapy,* 1991, vol. 45, (11): pp. 1007–14.

12 Elstein, A., Shulman, L. and Sprafka, A. *Medical Problem Solving.* Boston: Harvard University Press, 1978.

13 Cox, K. *Doctor and Patient.* Sydney: University of New South Wales Press, 1999.

14 Feinstein, A.R. An analysis of diagnostic reasoning, *Yale Journal of Biology and Medicine,* 1974, vol. 46, pp. 212–32.

15 Roter, D.L. and Hall, J.A. *Doctors Talking with Patients, Patients Talking with Doctors.* Westport, Conn.: Auburn House, 1992.

16 Balint, M. *The Doctor, His Patient and the Illness.* London: Pitman, 1964.

17 Hamrick, H.J. and Garfunkel, J.M. Clinical Decisions—how much analysis and how much judgement? *Journal of Paediatrics* 1991, vol. 118, p. 67.

8

Summaries and decisions

Catherine Berglund

The summary of information is a key part of health care. This chapter focuses on the summary of information as it is used with patients. Summary and briefing for other professionals is covered in more detail in a later chapter. The summary and checking of treatment expectations and the course of treatment that is planned is used as an example of summary both from patient to professional and professional to patient. Patient **decision-making**, or informed consent, is explored.

The summary and communication of information is a feature of health care, and the theme is obvious in many chapters in this book. In chapters 3 and 4 by Jill Gordon and Dimity Pond respectively, the concern is to capture, in summary form, how the patient feels, both physically and emotionally. In chapters that focus on communication between professionals, such as Elizabeth O'Brien's Chapter 10, 'Making a note and handover', and Max Kamien's Chapter 11, 'Good referral letters and good replies', the effective, concise summary of information about patient care is central. The willingness and availability of health care professionals and supporting mechanisms for the exchange of the summary is also crucial. In Chapter 13, 'Teams that work', interpersonal communication of objectives and summaries of options are the focus in stressful and demanding situations.

Each of these levels of summary and decision is part of the pursuit of care for the patient. This chapter illustrates the decision-making process, and its reliance on effective communication of information, as the patient makes informed decisions on treatment.

ELEMENTS OF NORMAL CONVERSATION AS PART OF INFORMATION EXCHANGE

The process of summary and exchange of information is essential in many forms of communication, just as it is between professionals, and between patients and professionals. In 'normal conversation', that is, normal communication exchange of oral form, the following elements should be present:

- conversational initiation: conversational responsiveness and participation
- turn-taking: cooperation in 'floor sharing'
- verbosity: perceived appropriateness of length of turn
- topic maintenance: relevance of contribution to topic in hand, and
- referencing: clarity in referring to people and events.[1]

These elements are expected for each participant in an active communication exchange. Once a 'normal' pattern is defined, it can serve as a template for assessing whether communication is adequate or not, or even whether it is inadequate to the point of being disordered. The focus of conversation is unique in a consultation, and may not involve equal interaction between parties, but elements of conversational interaction are still noticed by the participants.

Patient satisfaction with their physician is strongly communication dependent, as in the following survey items used by Terry and Healey. Their list represents the patient's perspective on the elements of successful active interaction. My doctor:

- spends enough time with me
- answers my questions
- listens to what I'm saying
- provides information so that I can make decisions about my care
- is concerned for me as a person as well as a patient
- explains things clearly
- reviews educational material with me.[2]

In some professional–patient interactions, the patient complains that he or she is not listened to. Could this be excessive turn-taking or verbosity by professionals? The issue of listening, without excessive interruption, was discussed by Jill Gordon in Chapter 3.

As well as voicing their own concerns and perspectives on their situation, patients need to give the professional significant conversation time, to relay relevant quality information that will be useful as they make decisions about what options in management and assessment to pursue. Professionals, in their conversations with patients, aim to achieve accuracy, efficiency, and supportiveness.[3]

In the elderly, particularly the 'older elderly', older than 75 years of age, certain conversational elements need to be facilitated to enhance effective communication. The older elderly have been found to be more likely to: be verbose; fail to maintain topic; have poor turn-taking skills; have unclear referencing in their conversations; and also to be less efficient in conveying descriptive information.[4] Much of the research to date has focused on the elderly patient. There is very little information on what these age-related changes in communication interaction mean for elderly practitioners.

COMPETENT DECISION-MAKING

The elements of adequate decision-making are routinely listed as:

- **competence** (ability to consent to what is being asked)
- information
- comprehension of that information
- voluntariness in making the decision, and
- reaching a decision.

Professionals have a key role in facilitating those elements. The health professional's task in informed decision-making, also called informed consent, is to listen to the concerns and information needs of the patient, and enable the patient to express those; and to provide the patient with information that is relevant and appropriate.

The elements of interaction in conversation outlined above appear to be crucial to the routine exchange of information in the process of consent. When conversation is not possible, or is not efficient, other methods for facilitating that exchange can be designed. When the people involved are from diverse cultural or language backgrounds, particular care needs to be taken in gathering information, exchanging information, and ensuring mutual understanding of issues and options. This was addressed in Chapter 2 by Dale Gietzelt and Gwyn Jones. For children, the provision of readily understood information is facilitated. There is also an ongoing assessment of what type of decision the child is ready to make as he or she becomes a 'mature minor'.[5]

There is, not surprisingly, additional effort in assessing the competence of elderly people to consent to medical treatment. Put simply, capacity interacts with the effectiveness of information exchanges. For patients making decisions about their own management and treatment, it is preferable to have the capacity to express themselves, and essential to have the capacity to hear and synthesise information from others, and to make reasoned decisions. The decision-making context has been a recognised focus of 'fitness to sign' **consent forms**, such as in the assessment suggested by Finucane et al. They have suggested that each of the following elements affects 'fitness to sign' in the elderly:

- conducive environment for decision-making
- cognitive function and stability over time
- functioning in activities of everyday living
- adequate information received and understood
- conducive frame of mind for decision-making
- health professional's conducive frame of mind
- family and social factors.[6]

INTEGRATING CONVERSATION, INFORMATION EXCHANGE, AND COMPETENCE

Table 8.1 integrates the elements of normal conversation with competence and comprehension concerns. The issues form a suggested checklist for conversations and information exchange between professionals and patients when the exchange is intended to lead to an informed decision on the part of the patient.

These steps may be worked through on more than one meeting. The process of information exchange in particular can be time consuming, and may naturally occur over a series of meetings to take into account developments in illness or health assessment, or further available options in management. Each decision may lead the health professional and patient to begin the steps anew, with different or more refined issues to be canvassed.

The segmentation of what is needed for effective communication in informed decision-making is consistent with thinking about communication as a series of learned skills. You could use the checklist to see what you are able to do well, and what you need to practise.

Initiation

The professional and the patient should share responsibility for the role in initiating the conversation, and raising issues of concern for exploration. This can be

Table 8.1: Competence and comprehension concerns in action

	Patient and professional can:
INITIATION	
Conducive context	Give proper time and attention for exchange
Conversational initiation	Raise and redirect to issues and concerns
INFORMATION EXCHANGE	
Turn-taking and verbosity	Listen without interrupting and hear other's input
Topic maintenance	Maintain depth in conversation
Referencing	Accurately relay clear and relevant input
SHARED UNDERSTANDING	
Adequate information	Revisit and weigh up information to hand
Comprehension	Exchange perception of what the other has said
DECISION	
Decision	Close conversation and express decision made

termed 'agenda setting'.[7] Each should feel able to add to the interaction with their concerns. A patient will be informed by their experiences, and a professional will be informed by what they observe in the patient, what they hear from the patient, and by their experience in dealing with similar issues.

The more difficult initiation for patients is in disclosure of personal matters. Rapport and trust are essential so that such areas may be discussed between professional and patient.

A notoriously difficult initiation for professionals is in the breaking of bad news. This is seen as an advanced communication skill, and can be learned gradually. Role-playing is useful in practising different ways of broaching the subject,[8] and then planning how to provide the necessary information to the patient.

Information exchange

The type of information that each brings to the exchange identifies the patient and the professional. For the patient, the information may be their life context, personal concerns, symptoms they have experienced, and individual preferences that would impact on the available options in management or treatment. This is to extend the agenda of treatment to 'take account of both disease and illness'.[9] The perspective of symptoms and the context of experiencing illness is recognised as being as informative as 'scientific' based enquiry to the traditional medical process of diagnosis and management.

For the professional, the information is the hallmark of their professional skill. It is gained from their assessment of the patient, in part, but also from their experience, and access to professional information resources. How the professional uses the information at his or her discretion is a difficult professional task. This has been a theme in preceding chapters. It is sufficient to note here that accessing professionally relevant information is a crucial first step to being part of an effective exchange with patients.

Although the information exchange is frequently achieved by conversation, it can be supplemented by written material. When written material is available, it is strongly suggested that each provider is familiar with that material, especially as the material can be sourced from many team members, the nurse, the clinician, or patient educator.[10] This makes good sense, as the patient may ask any of the providers about the issues covered in the material. It would become just one part of the information exchange between provider(s) and patient. When a patient sources information other than that provided, it is helpful to be able to discuss that information, its relevance and the patient's understanding of it. Tailoring the information the professional may provide for the patient and the context is another professional task. Each individual patient may want more, or less information, and may have different 'material' concerns. The gradual exchange of information is a process that blends in with further assessment, treatment, or management. It can be termed 'explanation and planning'.[11] The specific concerns of a patient about even remote risks may warrant additional information being provided under law.[12]

The tailoring of information is also tested in difficult clinical areas. In a recent editorial in a physiotherapy periodical, the importance of tailoring information on physical exercise for anorexic patients, who frequently adopt punishing exercise schedules, is described. The merit of including safe exercise, along with meditation and relaxation, is a current debate in the field. If exercise programs are to be advised, then access to relevant information held by all team members is essential in that process. An integrated understanding of the medical implications of advised programs, and the psychological implications are obviously crucial.[13] Team work and communication is the focus of Chapter 13, 'Teams that work'.

Shared understanding

The process of committed negotiation lends itself to shared responsibility for enhancing comprehension of each person's shared information and concerns. This process of checking that there is an understanding of the information to hand, the relevance of the information to the current medical situation, and the decision that lies ahead, is not just a check on the comprehension of the patient. It is also a check that appropriate understanding of the patient's perspective has been achieved by the professional.

To stop and check has also been termed 'chunking and checking'.[14] This is to summarise what has taken place in the interaction, and check mutual understanding of the issues at hand. It is an opportunity to re-enter the information exchange process, if it is needed, or if not, to go ahead to the decision-making step.

The commitment to the process of exchange and assessment of relevant information by both patient and professional is based on trust, and the process is founded on caring and concern.

Decision

The decision then becomes the result of the integrated communication interaction. There are choices about what decision-making model is appropriate. The choices are partly about who makes the decision about care. The model you prefer will impact on how you work through the preceding steps of initiation, information exchange, and shared understanding as well.

A paternalistic decision-making model is associated with the phrase 'Doctor knows best'. A paternalistic professional would care for the patient as a father would care for a child, and strive to make a decision (or suggest a decision to the patient) that would serve the patient's best interests. The decision on what may be 'best' is largely left to professional discretion.

The three other often-quoted decision-making models emphasise autonomy. Autonomy literally means self-rule, and the focus is on the patient making the decision about care processes.

An enhanced autonomy model allows for patients to decide what they would like, and that decision is 'enhanced' by the professional advice on what is professionally regarded as suitable or even best for the patient.[15] This is to allow autonomy, within a framework of professionally defined beneficence.

A model that allows for negotiation of primary concerns of care and self-rule has been suggested by Beauchamp and Childress. They suggested four principles of beneficence (obligation to care), non-maleficence (obligation to do no harm), autonomy (obligation to respect individuals and their wishes) and justice (obligation to fair distribution of resources) to be taken into account in health care interactions.[16] Each principle may be argued to be primary, if there is a conflict between obligations under them, depending on the people involved, the situation, and the context.

Under a libertarian model, each patient would choose what they wished, and their choice would be allowed as long as it did not significantly harm the similar liberties of others, nor threaten the 'fabric of society'.[17] This is to maximise each person's self-decision-making, according to their own notion of what is best for them.

These models are described further in ethics texts.[18] Decision-making is often emphasised in ethics, because of the high societal value placed on respect for individual wishes and personal integrity. Allowing and furthering the autonomy of a person is a basic way of respecting a person.

Other writers in the communication field have referred to decision models as the paternalistic model, and the consumeristic model, which correspond to the first and last models described above respectively. Another alternative is the *laissez-faire* model, in which no one accepts responsibility, and an aimless unproductive relationship results. The preferable model according to Silverman, Kurtz, and Draper is mutuality, in which active responsibility and negotiation are engaged in by patient and professional.[19] This model of mutuality seems closest to the model attributed to Beauchamp and Childress. If care from a professional perspective is emphasised in the mutual interaction, it could be regarded as equivalent to the enhanced autonomy model.

The more commonly adopted communication model in Western contexts is that of mutuality. As Streiffer and Nagle have stated in relation to patient education directed at patient behaviour change, '*together, physician and patient explore barriers to change, and negotiate achievable goals*', with the assistance of relevant '*knowledge-oriented patient education*'.[20]

The decision model adopted as acceptable practice is also an expression of the acceptable locus of control in the interaction.[21] In paternalism, least power is apparent in the patient. In libertarianism, most power is apparent. The subjective control over the health care process which is perceived by the patient has been studied extensively, as a factor in the progression of illness and recovery. It should be acknowledged, however, that not all patients prefer greater locus of control. The more recent picture of the patient is that there are at least two types: those people who are comfortable with deferring to expertise and delegating some power and responsibility to others, and those who prefer to feel in control of decisions themselves.[22] There are quite likely to be shades of preferences in between taking and deferring control. Some research indicates that there are patients who wish to be informed, but not to be actively involved in decision-making.[23] There are well-documented cultural differences in being told the truth and making one's own decisions.[24] Perhaps the locus of control is as negotiable as the type and amount of information which is exchanged.

INTERACTION

The readiness of both patient and professional to engage in relevant information exchange, and discussion is crucial to the success of the interaction.

For patients, there is a routine assessment of capacity to make certain decisions, and there is a commitment on the part of health professionals to facilitate the actual decision by provision of relevant information and the maximisation of a conducive environment. Substitute decision-makers can be used, such as guardianship system, if needed.

The facilitation of the interaction depends on the competence and readiness of the health care professional as much as on the competence and decision-making readiness of the patient. A highly skilled professional will have better quality assessment and resulting synthesised information ready for the patient. A health professional who is a highly skilled communicator will be able to make that summary and synthesis accessible for patients in their decision-making process. Figure 8.1 illustrates how dependent the patient is on the input of the competent professional to be not only ready but also able to make an adequate informed decision on their own health care.

The complexity of skill required for the professional to be an effective partner in decision-making with the patient should not be underestimated. It could draw on skills that are as diverse as: building trust and rapport with the patient; the gathering of patient information in direct observation and enquiry of the patient; the sourcing of relevant professional knowledge, and other professionals' advice and experience; the synthesis and analysis of information from a

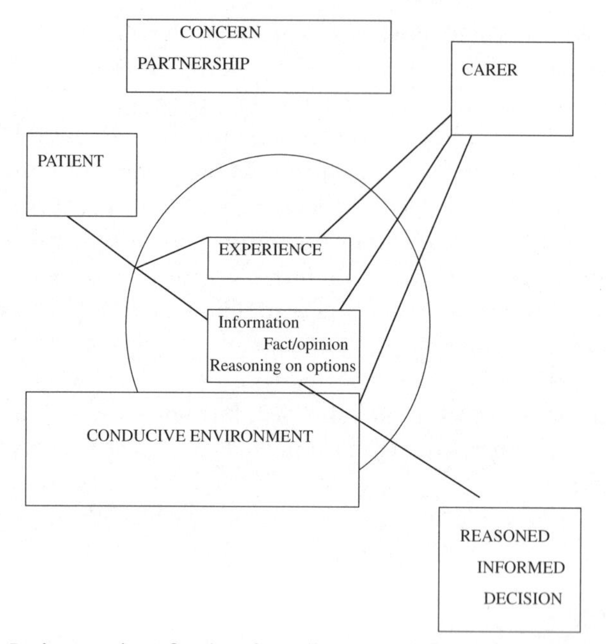

Figure 8.1 Patient and professional readiness for informed decision-making

number of sources; the effective summary of that information; effective use of team discussions; and assessment of personal ability in performance of technical procedures.

The key purpose of the interaction is care. A joint concern for the continued care of the patient is the foundation for an interaction. This requires the effort of both parties, as represented in Figure 8.1. Ideally, both parties can trust to divulge and exchange information, and explore issues in assessment, management, and treatment.

The process of health professionals negotiating reasonable options and advice for their patients is of course undertaken within a broad cultural and social context. The compatibility of the organisational structures, which the health professionals work in, with social contexts is crucial to the success of initiatives from those health professionals.[25] Some writers term the interaction between patient and professional a 'transaction'.[26] This also acknowledges the broader social context of each interaction and decision in health care.

NOTES

1 Mackenzie, C. Adult spoken discourse: The influences of age and education, *International Journal of Language and Communication Discourse,* 2000, vol. 35, no. 2, pp. 269–85, p. 273.

2 Terry, P.E. and Healey, M.L. The physician's role in educating patients: a comparison of mailed versus physician-delivered patient education, *The Journal of Family Practice,* 2000, vol. 49, no. 4, pp. 314–18, p. 317.
3 Kurtz, S., Silverman, J., and Draper, J. *Teaching and Learning Communication Skills in Medicine.* Radcliffe Medical Press, Abingdon, Oxon, 1998, p. 29.
4 Mackenzie, C. Adult spoken discourse: the influences of age and education, *International Journal of Language and Communication Discourse,* 2000, vol. 35, no. 2, pp. 269–85, p. 279.
5 Berglund, C.A. and Devereux, J.A. Consent to medical treatment: Children making medical decisions for others, *Australian Journal of Forensic Sciences,* 2000, vol. 32, pp. 25–36.
6 Finucane, P., Myser, C. and Ticehurst, S. 'Is she fit to sign Doctor?': Practical ethical issues in assessing the competence of elderly patients, *Medical Journal of Australia*, 1993, vol. 159, no. 6, pp. 400–3, p. 402.
7 Silverman, J., Kurtz, S. and Draper, J. *Skills for Communicating with Patients.* Radcliffe Medical Press, Abingdon, Oxon, 1998, p. 33.
8 Kurtz, S., Silverman, J. and Draper, J. *Teaching and Learning Communication Skills in Medicine*, p. 144.
9 Silverman, J., Kurtz, S. and Draper, J. *Skills for Communicating with Patients*, p. 40.
10 McVea, K.L.S.P., Venugopal, M., Crabtree, B.F. and Aita, V. The organization and distribution of patient education materials in family medicine practices, *The Journal of Family Practice,* 2000, vol. 49, no. 4, pp. 319–26, p. 322.
11 Silverman, J., Kurtz, S. and Draper, J. *Skills for Communicating with Patients*, p. 100.
12 For instance, the High Court decision in Australia, *Rogers v. Whitaker* (1992) 175 CLR 479.
13 Editorial. Tackling the twin faces of Anorexia: physiotherapy's role in helping sufferers correct distorted body images, *Frontline*, 2000, March 15, pp.10–11.
14 Silverman, J., Kurtz, S. and Draper, J. *Skills For Communicating With Patients*, p. 100.
15 Quill, T.E. and Brody, H. Physician recommendations and patient autonomy: Finding a balance between physician power and patient choice. *Annals of Internal Medicine*, 1996, vol. 125, no. 9, pp. 763–9.
16 Beauchamp, T.L. and Childress, J.F. *Principles of Biomedical Ethics.* 4th edn, Oxford University Press, New York, 1994.
17 Mill, J.S. On liberty, in J.S. Mill. *Three Essays.* Oxford University Press, London, 1975 (first published 1859).
18 Berglund, C.A. *Ethics for Health Care.* Oxford University Press, Melbourne, 1998.
19 Silverman, J., Kurtz, S. and Draper, J. *Skills for Communicating with Patients*, p. 116.
20 Streiffer, R.H. and Nagle, J.P. Patient education in our offices, *The Journal of Family Practice,* 2000, vol. 49, no. 4, pp. 327–8, p. 328.
21 Northouse, L.L. and Northouse, P.G. *Health Communication: Strategies for Health Professionals.* Appleton & Lange, Stamford, Conn., 1998, p. 35.
22 de Ridder, D., Depla, M., Severens, P. and Malsch, M. Beliefs on Coping with Illness: A Consumer's Perspective, *Social Science & Medicine,* 1997, vol. 44, no. 5, pp. 553–9.

23 Deber, R.B., Kraetschmer, N. and Irvine, J. What role do patients wish to play in treatment decision making? *Archives of Internal Medicine,* 1996, vol. 156, pp. 1414–20.
24 Surbone, A. and Zwitter, M. (eds). Communication with the Cancer Patient: Information & Truth, *Annals of the New York Academy of Sciences* 1997, vol. 809, New York Academy of Sciences, New York.
25 Skold, P. The key to success: The role of local government in the organization of smallpox vaccination in Sweden, *Medical History,* 2000, vol. 45, pp. 201–26, p. 222.
26 Northouse, L.L. and Northouse, P.G. *Health Communication: Strategies for Health Professionals*, p. 19.

9

Consultations and interactions

Natalie O'Dea and Deborah Saltman

The interaction between a clinician and a patient can be seen as a meeting of experts. The clinician has specialised knowledge about health care and the patient has specialised knowledge and insight about themselves.[1] During the consultation, knowledge transfer takes place and together the clinician and the patient can make a therapeutic interaction occur. To date, the ongoing relationship between clinician and patient has been viewed as a series of discrete interactions. In the future, the impact of multiple co-morbidities on patient outcomes will mean that the clinical focus will shift from acute results achieved in one consultation to long-term health management strategies over a series of consultations.

This chapter explores the interactions between clinician and patient, focusing on a patient learning new health management strategies with the assistance of a clinician. We describe a model called Situational Leadership (SL II), which can be used in the ongoing relationship between a patient and a clinician. The model looks at the development stages a patient goes through when learning a new task, such as their role in the management of their illness. The corresponding leadership styles that the clinician can adopt to help their patient learn new tasks are also delineated in the model.

To describe this model, we have chosen the task of learning how to drive a car. The application of the model to a clinical setting will then be shown through the example of an obese patient learning weight management strategies. The desired outcome will be to assist a patient to learn how to achieve and maintain the 'task' of healthy weight.[2] Through this difficult-to-manage clinical scenario, we will explore how the model can be applied throughout a series of consultations.

THE SITUATIONAL LEADERSHIP II MODEL

The Situational Leadership II model (SL II model), described by Blanchard in 1985, is used widely in management circles to assist leaders develop their team members' skills.[3] This model is based on the premise that team members/learners go through a series of stages on the way to learning a new task. The learner's development stage is then matched with an appropriate leadership style by the leader. The process of identifying the development stage of a learner and then using the appropriate leadership style to assist the learner are the two key features of this model.

DEVELOPMENT STAGES

A learner goes through four development stages (D) in the process of mastering a new task. They are:

- D1 = Enthusiastic beginner
- D2 = Disenchanted learner
- D3 = Capable but cautious performer
- D4 = Self-reliant achiever.

In each of these stages, the two main factors that affect the development level of the learner are:

- Competence, which encompasses their level of knowledge and skill
- Commitment, which encompasses their degree of confidence and motivation.

Competence and commitment fluctuate throughout the learning process. The four development stages as outlined in the model will be illustrated through the task of learning how to drive a car.

Development Stage 1 (D1)—the 'enthusiastic beginner'

D1—the 'enthusiastic beginner'—displays the characteristics of:

- High commitment: 'I really want to be able to drive a car.'
- Low competence: 'I don't know how to drive, but I'm ready to learn.'

The D1—'enthusiastic beginner'—is ready and willing to perform the task such as driving a car, but has limited understanding of how to do it. When a person is ready to get their learner's permit to drive a car, the level of competence in driving is very low. The skill or knowledge necessary to drive a car is absent. On the other hand, the 'enthusiastic beginner' is usually highly committed and highly motivated to learn how to drive and therefore full of confidence that they can join the millions of other motorists on the road. Such a learner is deemed 'unconsciously incompetent'.

D1—the 'enthusiastic beginner'—needs:

- Clear goals: 'Today we are going to learn how to reverse-park.'
- Standards: 'You need to stay in one lane, the lines marked will help you do this.'
- 'Hands-on' training: 'Let's try that hill start again.'
- Frequent feedback: 'Slow down. You are going well, just don't go so fast.'
- Recognition of enthusiasm: 'It's great that you want to learn how to drive.'

Development Stage 2 (D2)—the 'disenchanted learner'

D2—the 'disenchanted learner' —displays the characteristics of:

- Low commitment: 'It's too hard to learn how to drive, I just can't do it.'
- Low to some competence: 'I can steer the car, but I'm not sure how to reverse-park. Driving is not as easy as I thought it would be.'

As knowledge and skill increase, the learner may find out just how much remains to be learnt. They become 'consciously incompetent' and may struggle with the enormity of the task. The 'disenchanted learner' not only has limited skills, but also has probably had a few setbacks and has lost some of the motivation and confidence necessary to achieve task-mastery.

With our driving analogy, once the learner starts lessons, it may soon become apparent that there is more to driving than meets the eye. It may be difficult to turn tight corners, hard to keep the car on the correct side of the road and the windscreen wipers may be mistaken for the indicator. The learner's competence has increased slightly; however, commitment usually drops as it becomes clear that the task may not be as simple as it first seemed. The learner becomes disenchanted. This stage is often called the 'too hard basket' and may result in the learner giving in, saying that the task will never be mastered, in this case: 'I will never be able to drive a car, it's too hard. I'll just keep on taking public transport.'

D2—the 'disillusioned learner'—needs:

- Perspective and explanations of why: 'Drive slower in the rain because you are more likely to skid in wet conditions.'
- Frequent feedback on results: 'Well done, you are parking much closer to the curb now.'
- Assurance that it is OK to make mistakes: 'It doesn't matter if you hit the curb, try again.'
- Involvement in decision-making: 'Do you want to practise some more reverse-parking?'
- Encouragement and praise for making progress: 'That was a very good lesson. You have certainly improved.'

Development Stage 3 (D3)—the 'capable but cautious performer'

D3—the 'capable but cautious performer'—displays the characteristics of:

- Variable commitment: 'Most of the time I am comfortable driving. I just don't like those rainy nights.'
- Moderate to high competence: 'I know enough to pass the test, but I still hesitate at busy intersections.'

In this development stage, while a moderate to high degree of competence has been achieved, confidence and motivation may still be labile. Setbacks at this time for the D3—'capable but cautious performer'—will have large effects on confidence, although most of the knowledge and skills to complete the task have been acquired. At this stage the learner is 'consciously competent'.

In our driving example, after a few more lessons, and perhaps some near misses, the learner's competence has increased and essentially they know how to handle a car. Although skill and knowledge have increased, the learner's confidence and motivation waivers. Driving at night, in heavy rain, or on country roads may seem a bit daunting. The learner at this point may need more practice and reassurance.

D3—the 'capable but cautious performer'—needs:

- An approachable **mentor** or **coach**: 'Is there anything else you would like to practise?'
- Opportunities to express concerns: 'You are right to be worried about drinking and driving. How much do you think you can drink before you reach the limit?'
- Support and encouragement to develop problem-solving skills: 'You now know how to check the oil and water. How would you prepare the car before taking a long trip?'
- Help in looking at skills objectively so confidence is built: 'You have been through the driving test checklist and you can do all the components. You are ready to go for your licence.'
- Praise and recognition for good performance: 'Good driving. You slowed down well in advance of that pedestrian crossing.'

Development Stage 4 (D4)—the 'self-reliant achiever'

D4—the 'self-reliant achiever'—displays the characteristics of:

- High commitment: 'I like the freedom driving gives me.'
- High competence: 'I'm a very good driver with an impeccable record.'

The D4—'self-reliant achiever'—stage is the aim of every learner and leader. The learner has the necessary competence and commitment for task accomplishment and is 'unconsciously competent'.

Here we have the 'Gold Licence Driver', highly competent in their skill and knowledge about driving. They are also highly committed, with the motivation and confidence to continue driving. This driver can now teach somebody else how to drive.

D4—the 'self-reliant achiever'—needs:

- Variety and challenge: 'You seem ready for the advanced driving course.'
- Trust: 'You are a good driver—can you teach your brother to drive?'
- A leader who is more a mentor and colleague than a 'boss': 'Call me if you ever need help with the car.'
- Acknowledgment of contributions: 'Thanks for driving me to work every day.'

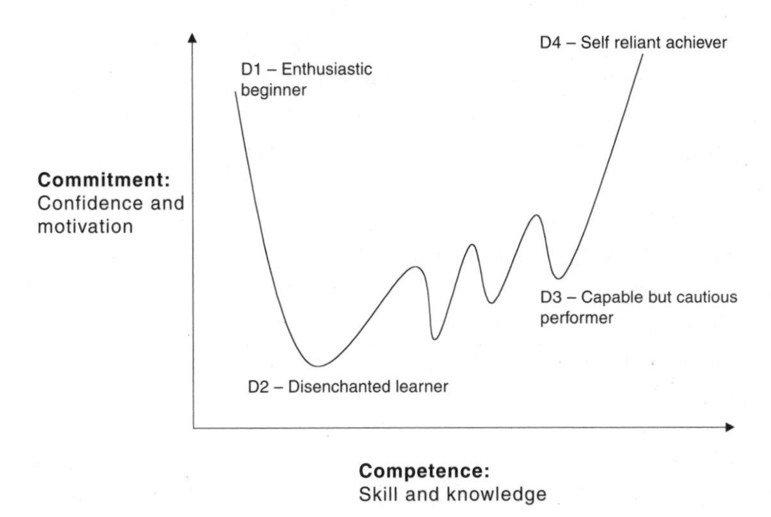

Figure 9.1 Development stages

- Autonomy and authority: 'You can drive my car whenever I am not using it.' The developmental stages are displayed diagrammatically in Figure 9.1.

RECOGNISING LEARNER LEVELS

The progression from D1—'enthusiastic beginner'—to D4—'self-reliant achiever'—may not be smooth, or always in the direction towards D4. Learners may experience problems along the way that send them backwards rather than forward along the path. For example, in our driving analogy, a D3—'capable but cautious performer'—who is involved in a car accident may slide back to the D2—'disenchanted learner'—stage.

LEADERSHIP STYLES

The first part of the model, which has been described, deals with diagnosing the development stage of the learner. In the second part of the model, we look at how leadership styles change according to this diagnosis. In the model, a leader displays four leadership styles (S). They are:

- S1 = Directing
- S2 = Coaching
- S3 = Supporting
- S4 = Delegating

In each of these styles the two main factors that determine the leadership style of a leader are:

- the level of direction given to the learner (directive leadership)
- the level of support given to the learner (supportive leadership).

Directive leadership behaviour is task-focused. It is when a leader:

- provides structure
- organises the task
- instructs and explains how to do the task
- supervises the conduct of the task.

Supportive leadership behaviour is relationship-focused. It is when a leader:

- provides encouragement and praise
- listens and empathises
- facilitates discussion
- gives perspective and assurance.

The four leadership styles (S1, S2, S3, S4) correspond to the four development levels (D1, D2, D3, D4) of the learner (see Figure 9.2). Continuing with our analogy of learning how to drive a car, here is an overview of how each of the leadership styles applies to the corresponding development stage of a learner.

D1: Enthusiastic beginner High commitment Low competence 'Unconsciously incompetent' **D1 – S1** **S1: Directing leadership** High direction Low support 'I'll decide'	**D2: Disenchanted learner** Low commitment Low to fair competence 'Consciously incompetent' **D2 – S2** **S2: Coaching leadership** High direction High support 'We'll talk, I'll decide'
D3: Capable but cautious performer Variable commitment Moderate to high competence 'Consciously competent' **D3 – S3** **S3: Supporting leadership** Low direction High support 'We'll talk, you'll decide'	**D4: Self-reliant achiever** High commitment High competence 'Unconsciously competent' **D4 – S4** **S4: Delegating leadership** Low direction Low support 'You decide'

Figure 9.2 Situational Leadership II

Situational Leadership Style 1 (S1)—'directing'

S1—'directing' leadership—displays the characteristics of:

- high direction
- low support.

The S1—'directing' leadership style is used with a learner in D1—'enthusiastic beginner'. It is the most task-focused style of leadership. As a beginner has low competence, the leader needs to give a lot of direction.

Using our driving analogy, statements such as 'this is how you put the key in the ignition, this is the way you turn the key' and 'this pedal is the brake, that other pedal is the accelerator' could be used. As the learner is enthusiastic, full of confidence and motivation, the leader does not need to be supportive. At this stage a lot of direction provided by the leader will in fact be received as supportive, as direction is what the learner needs to feel supported in their learning process.

The language of the highly directive leadership style is very specific. Sentences are short and to the point to allow for the transmission of clear messages. The focus of the sentences is on what the learner should do. There is little room for discussion or exploration of issues. As the D1—'enthusiastic beginner's'—motivation is high, there is little need for reinforcing or motivating statements.

S1—'directing'—leadership actions include:

- outlining clear standards, goals, and boundaries
- providing 'hands-on' training
- recognising enthusiasm
- giving frequent feedback.

Leadership Style 2 (S2)—'coaching'

S2—'coaching'—leadership displays the characteristics of:

- high direction
- high support.

The S2—'coaching'—leadership style is the most time consuming, and matches with the D2—'disenchanted learner'—who may be ready to give up. This leadership style is characterised by high direction and high support. When teaching someone how to drive a car, statements such as '*It's OK, I've got my hand on the brake. Just keep your eyes on the road, slow down, put your indicator on*' and '*You are doing just fine*' may be used. The leader 'coaches' the learner to increase all of their components: skill, knowledge, confidence, and motivation.

The language of highly directive and highly supportive communication is more conversational. There is an emphasis on the partnership between the learner and the leader. However, this emphasis on the partnership between the two relies on the leader maintaining the role of senior partner. 'We' and 'let us see' are used more often to signify this partnership. However, the overall message is clear, the D2—'disenchanted learner'—must be provided with knowledge and skills through direction, and motivation and confidence through support.

S2—'coaching'—leadership actions include:

- encouraging involvement in decision-making
- praising progress and providing encouragement
- providing perspective and explanations of why
- assuring that it is OK to make mistakes.

Leadership Style 3 (S3)—'supporting'

S3—'supporting'—leadership displays the characteristics of:

- low direction
- high support.

The S3—'supporting'—leadership style matches with the D3—'capable but cautious performer'. This style is low in direction as the learner knows how to do the task, but high in support as the learner's confidence and motivation waivers. In our driving analogy encouragement and feedback on driving technique are needed. Statements such as 'You are really driving well. I feel very comfortable as your passenger' could be used. In this way, the learner will feel reassured by an extra set of eyes on the road.

The language of the low directive and high supportive leadership style is also conversational. However, the emphasis of the partnership between the learner and leader is on the learner adopting the role of senior partner. 'We' and 'let us see' are replaced with 'you decide' and 'you can do it' more often, to signify this change in the partnership. The D3—'capable but cautious performer'—needs to assume more responsibility for their own task-mastery with some support available from the leader.

S3—'supporting'—leadership actions include:

- mentoring or coaching
- helping to look at skills objectively so confidence is built
- praising and recognising good performance
- supporting and encouraging the development of problem-solving skills.

Leadership Style 4 (S4)—'delegating'

S4—'delegating' leadership displays the characteristics of:

- low direction
- low support.

The S4—'delegating'—leadership style is the least time consuming as the D4—'self-reliant achiever'—does not need a lot of direction nor support. The 'learner' knows how to perform the task. They can also deal with problems if necessary. In our car analogy, it is the time when the car keys are handed over with confidence: 'Feel free to use my car.'

The language of the low directive and low supportive leadership style is less discursive. There is an emphasis on the learner's autonomy, not the partnership. The D4—'self reliant achiever'—has assumed responsibility for their continued task-mastery. 'You decide' and 'you can do it' are replaced with 'let me know if you need me'.

S4—'delegating'—leadership actions include:

- allowing for autonomy and authority
- acknowledging contributions
- supporting variety and challenge
- trusting.

In summary, the skills of a good situational leader include:

- The ability to recognise and diagnose the development stage of the learner.
- The flexibility to change leadership style according to the needs of the learner.
- The capacity to form an effective relationship/partnership with the learner.

SITUATIONAL LEADERSHIP II MODEL IN CLINICAL PRACTICE

Communication with patients about complex, chronic conditions that are often relapsing can prove to be a special challenge. The SL II model can provide health care professionals with a framework to assist them in communicating with their patients over a series of consultations to achieve specific tasks.

All patients respond to a communication style that works for them in a particular situation. An effective health care professional can recognise the needs of the patient and is flexible enough to match their style to the needs of the patient. Just as the driving analogy was used to describe the model, the task of achieving healthy weight will show how this model works in the communication over time between clinician and patient.

Development Stage 1 (D1)—the 'enthusiastic beginner' patient

When the obese patient arrives for a consultation, because they have come to see the clinician, we assume there is already a certain level of motivation present to initiate a learning pathway. This D1—'enthusiastic beginner'—may be confident and/or motivated to lose weight, but does not have the skill or knowledge to best achieve this goal. The D1—'enthusiastic beginner'—has experienced positive or negative motivators that have given them the impetus to embark on a weight loss program. Examples of positive motivators may include new weight reduction therapies available, supportive partners or pleasurable events in the future. Negative motivators may include serious health consequences of obesity such as diabetes or hypertension, or a need to escape the social stigma of obesity.

This is the point where an obese patient may resolve to 'go on a diet', but their knowledge about such a process is lacking. With increased knowledge facilitated by the clinician, the patient could be moved to talk about lifestyle changes rather than just 'diet'. At this development stage, the enthusiasm of the patient needs to be harnessed and directed.

Statements that provide clues that a patient may be in the D1—'enthusiastic beginner'—stage in relation to their weight management include:

- 'I would really like to lose weight, but I don't know why I can't—I don't have any fat in my diet.'
- 'My mother had a bypass last week. I think it's time I started getting serious about my own health.'
- 'I've tried a lot of things in the past, but I guess this approach could be different …'
- 'Now that summer is almost over, I think I can start exercising.'
- 'My friend told me that you know ways of helping to increase her exercise that are easy and not like going to the gym.'
- 'I've heard you prescribe this new tablet that can really help me to lose weight—can I try it?'

Situational Leadership Style 1 (S1)—'directing' clinician

Patients who are highly motivated and confident need little support. In the first of a series of consultations focused on achieving a task such as weight loss, a patient may be motivated but does not know how to proceed. They will need a lot of direction.

Here are some statements that an S1—'directing'—clinician may make in relation to a D1 patient on a weight management program:

- 'Let's aim for you to lose 9kg in the next nine months.'
- 'In the next four months, let's aim to reduce your clothes size by two.'
- 'Initially, come and see me every three weeks.'
- 'Take one capsule within an hour of eating (before or after meals).'
- 'For starters, walk for approximately 15 minutes three times a week.'
- 'Enrol in the weight management program.'
- 'Eat less than 40 grams of fat. Here is a menu planner.'
- 'It's great that you want to lose weight, now let's talk about how.'
- 'Here is some information for you take away and read. Next time we will discuss it.'

Development Stage 2 (D2)—the 'disenchanted learner' patient

The obese patient attempting to lose weight may become disenchanted when they realise weight loss does not happen quickly, and it requires a long-term effort. Their knowledge and skill in relation to weight loss has slightly increased, but effective weight management is not yet mastered. The increased amount of knowledge may lead to a fall in confidence and motivation when the patient realises just how much is involved. This is the point where most weight loss programs are abandoned.

The obese patient who has made several previous attempts with limited success may start this series of consultations as a D2—'disenchanted learner'—rather than D1—'enthusiastic beginner'. Patients whose weight loss has plateaued or who have put on weight will also exhibit patterns of communication in a subsequent consultation that may suggest they are also a disenchanted learner. Statements that a D2—'disenchanted learner'—may make in relation to their weight management include:

- 'I've tried absolutely everything before. Nothing works.'
- 'Everyone at home eats the same things. I just can't change my diet.'
- 'I've had home-delivered meals, I even tried not eating—I just can't seem to lose weight.'
- 'All my family are fat. It's just impossible—it's in my genes.'
- 'I just can't diet, and exercise makes me hot and sweaty.'
- 'I was never any good at this goal-setting business.'
- 'I am sorry that I disappointed you.'
- 'I started out with good intentions, I just can't stick to it. I feel so bad.'

Leadership Style 2 (S2)—'coaching' clinician

Examples of the type of highly directive and highly supportive language that can assist communication with a patient trying to master the task of weight loss, but who has lost motivation and confidence include:

- 'You can lose weight, you've done it before. Let's work out how we can keep it off this time.'
- 'Nuts are high in protein, but they also have a lot of fat, perhaps we can plan some low-fat snacks together.'
- 'Although you haven't lost as much weight as you wanted to, it's great that you've lost three centimetres from around your waist.'
- 'Remember that your weight loss will reduce your health risks significantly.'
- 'I'm pleased you've come back to see me. I'm here to support you. Let's see who else can provide some support.'
- 'If you think it's too cold and dark in the morning to go walking, perhaps you can walk at lunchtime.'
- 'Let's go through the information you received from the weight management program and discuss any issues that came up for you.'

Development Stage 3 (D3)—the 'capable but cautious performer' patient

The D3—'capable but cautious performer'—knows the necessary steps and has the competence to successfully lose weight, but has wavering motivation and confidence in the ability to do so. This patient will need to focus on the small successes along the way to maintain commitment to the process. The patient knows the 'right' things to do for weight loss, but may not always want to do them.

Once the obese patient has succeeded in losing weight or achieving another indicator, such as looser clothes fit, they are well on the way to competent task-mastery. Statements that a D3—'capable but cautious performer'—may make in relation to their weight management include:

- 'I know what I have to do, but nobody supports me at home.'
- 'My weight loss has plateaued—what can I do about it?'
- 'It really helps to have someone at the end of the telephone to talk to.'
- 'Some days it's so hard; other days I don't even have to think about it.'
- 'My pedometer provides me with the encouragement I need to keep walking every day.'
- 'I guess if I can focus on what is achievable every week, I don't have to worry about setbacks so much.'

Situational Leadership Style 3 (S3)—'supportive' clinician

The D3—'capable but cautious performer'—will require support (the level of which will vary) but little direction, as they know how to lose weight and keep it off. However, sometimes problems arise and they need a little more support to stop them sliding back into the D2—'disenchanted learner'. Examples of the type of language that can assist communication with a patient trying to maintain motivation and confidence during the task of weight loss include:

- 'I can see from your food diary that you can prepare low fat meals. How do you think you can make this second nature?'
- 'Well done, it's been three months and you've lost three kilograms. What obstacles do you see ahead in the next three months?'
- 'I can understand why you are having difficulty maintaining your activity schedule because of your work commitments. Do you have any ideas about how to get around this?'
- 'You've plateaued before and succeeded in losing weight. What additional resources do you think you need this time?'
- 'You are right, you know how to keep the weight off. However, it's natural that your motivation will wax and wane.'

Development Stage 4 (D4)—the 'self-reliant achiever'

The D4—'self-reliant achiever'—has successfully lost weight and has the commitment to keep it off. Skills, knowledge, motivation, and confidence are all high. This is the learning stage that obese patients aiming to lose weight would like to maintain.

Statements that a D4—'self-reliant achiever' —may make in relation to their weight management include:

- 'I have worked out how to cook low fat meals that all the family can enjoy.'
- 'The tablets certainly kept me on track with what food I should and shouldn't eat—now I know which foods to avoid.'
- 'My clothes size has dropped by two sizes and I feel fantastic.'
- 'I have just come to tell you that I have achieved yet another of my goals—thank you.'

Situational Leadership Style 4 (S4)—'delegating' clinician

The D4—'self-reliant achiever'—requires little support and little direction. They know how to lose weight and keep it off. Examples of the type of language that can assist communication with a patient who has achieved committed and competent task-mastery include:

- 'Congratulations for maintaining your healthy weight target.'
- 'You know the warning signals that tell you when you lose motivation and confidence and subsequently gain weight. If that happens, come and see me.'
- 'It's been two months since you stopped taking the tablets and you've maintained your weight loss, you are obviously eating the right foods and keeping up your physical activity.'
- 'What are your plans to keep your healthy weight over the next twelve months?'

CONCLUSION

Not all health problems are easily translated into tasks that both the clinician and the patient can agree upon. For example, a general practitioner may want to deal with a patient's obesity while the patient may only want a 'quick fix' through tablets to treat the hypertension that is a consequence of the obesity. In such cases, mismatches or ill-defined tasks can be 'bookmarked' for review at a later date. Whatever task is identified in a consultation as significant, both clinician and patient will need to agree on it and work out an ongoing strategy to achieve a healthy outcome.

Sustainable impact is the key long-term outcome in an ongoing relationship between clinician and patient. Although often comprising a series of short-term successes, long-term change is much more significant than any one short-term gain. Using long-term strategies such as SL II, clinicians have the opportunity to partner with their patients over a number of consultations to achieve a successful health outcome. Consultation style, where a task is to be mastered, depends on the development stage of the patient (learner), the corresponding leadership style of the clinician (leader), as well as the consultation issues to be dealt with. The model emphasises that the scope to direct and support change within a series of consultations is dependent on achieving the appropriate style of communication and leadership at each consultation along the way.

Flexibility is an essential skill in adopting situationally appropriate leadership styles. Research into the application of the Situational Leadership II Model in Australia shows that most leaders have a preference for one leadership style over the other. Australian usage of SL II reveals that 51 per cent of managers use only one style comfortably; 30 per cent of this population use two styles comfortably; 18 per cent use three styles comfortably; and only 1 per cent of the management population use all four styles comfortably.[4]

A health consultation may be more conducive to the use of all four leadership styles due to its inherent flexibility. Clinicians are used to altering their style according to the nature of the consultation. For example, where a patient is suffering from an acute life-threatening emergency such as an exacerbation of heart failure, there is less scope for meaningful verbal exchange.[5] The interaction between clinician and patient would be very direct. Whereas a subsequent check up, which is the most frequent reason for encounter with a general practitioner, may be more collaborative.[6]

When applied to a consultation, the SL II model may enhance communication between clinician and patient. The clinician, using the SL II model, can identify the needs of the patient; match the appropriate leadership style; monitor the progression of the patient in mastering a health task; and thereby improve the patient's health outcome.

NOTES

1 Tuckett, D. *Meetings Between Experts: An Approach to Sharing Ideas in Medical Consultations.* 1985, Tavistock, New York.

2 Blanchard, K., Zigarmi, D. and Zigarmi, P. *Situational Leadership II. Facilitator Guide.* 1994, Blanchard Training and Development Inc., CA.

3 Blanchard, K. *Situational Leadership: The Colour Model.* 1995, Blanchard Training and Development Inc., CA.

4 Professional Training and Development Group. 2000. Sydney (personal communication).

5 Saltman, D.C. and O'Dea, N.A. General practice consultations: Quality time? *Medical Journal of Australia*, 1999, vol. 171, p. 76.

6 Bridges-Webb, C., Britt, H., Miles, D.A., Neary, S., Charles, J. and Traynor, V. Morbidity and treatment in general practice in Australia 1990–1991, *Medical Journal of Australia*, 1992, vol. 157 Suppl., S22–4.

10

Making a note and handover

Elizabeth O'Brien

For all health care workers, continuity of patient care depends on coordinated and integrated patient management. Central to this process is the interaction between providers who are involved in patient care. Communication links providers to patients and to each other.[1] This chapter is written from a nursing perspective. The messages are relevant for all health care professionals. The making of notes is a fundamental communication exercise in health care. Notes often form the basis for further communication between team members, and across time in dealing with patients. Two particular interactive communication processes, essential for continuity of care, in which nurses are involved, are handover and referral. These processes are important, especially within the context of a changing health care system.

A number of factors have changed and continue to change the delivery of health care in Australia; these challenge continuity of care, particularly in a nursing context. These changes include:[2]

1 Changed clinical practices, due to new technology and pharmacology. For example, where once a particular procedure required a seven-day hospital stay, with the use of keyhole surgery it requires a one-day stay. Another example is the ability to deliver intravenous antibiotics in the home setting of patients, rather than in hospital.
2 Changed hospital and treatment practices, where hospitals are becoming increasingly specialised and are only one component of a broader health system. A patient will often receive services from a number of providers in a number of settings for one illness episode or incident. Once hospitals provided all aspects of care from the onset of the problem or treatment to recovery. Now many services are provided in the community from pre-admission and post-acute care to long-term care.
3 Budgetary constraints may be seen as the most important factor of change responsible for changed work practices. These have resulted in: decreased length of stay for patients; increased use of casual staff; changed shift lengths

(some longer, some shorter); decreased time of staff changeover; higher staff turnover and the increasing use of nursing assistants.

Nurses may be seen as central to the process of continuing care and therefore should be equipped with the communication skills and processes to manage care within a complicated and somewhat fragmented health care system. Handover and referral practices have been greatly affected by the above changes over recent years, as they are central to ensuring effective and continuing care.

NOTES AS A BASIS FOR COMMUNICATION

In order to provide effective and efficient care, health care providers must communicate with each other. The institutions or organisations in which the health providers work must provide the framework and systems to enable processes of effective and efficient communication, both within their own organisation and between organisations.

Due to the scale of change in all areas of health service delivery, the use of documentation to support communication has increased. Both patient handover and referral must be supported by excellent documentation. Documentation performs a number of important functions in terms of communication. It:[3]

1 promotes communication among staff;
2 ensures a total, sequential overview of patient care;
3 avoids duplication of information;
4 ensures consistency of care; and
5 guards against the loss of information.

Documentation also functions to provide:

- data for research and review of services;
- evidence of work practices for funding purposes; and
- evidence of care for legal purposes.

It is therefore important to briefly describe the ways in which nurses document the care given and care planned for patients, prior to discussing handover and referral.

In the past, nurses documented the 'medical' care they provided, but were entrenched in an 'oral tradition' where *'they write what they must to keep out of trouble, but pass on "real" information verbally'.*[4] Now, it is important for nurses to document the 'real' information to ensure continuity of care within the current health care climate. Well-planned and concise documentation is an essential element of continuity of care.

The format of documentation by nurses has gone through many transitions, as the health system has changed. There was a time when nursing notes were not included in the patient progress notes. When they were then included, they were stored in a separate section of the notes. Following this, they were included in the general progress notes, but may have been written in different coloured ink. They were more than likely overlooked by other health care providers. The separation of nursing from medical and other health provider notes only served to create and maintain barriers to the effective flow of information about patients. Now, in general, a single health record is used, in which all providers involved in care of the patient write.

Nurses record information in a number of important documents. These include (among others): patient progress notes (health/patient record); **nursing care plans**; treatment charts; and observation charts. Over the last ten years, documentation requirements have increased to the extent that a large proportion of nurses' time is spent with documentation compliance at the expense of 'hands on' patient care. Attempts are now made to streamline documentation, making it more concise and less time-consuming while reducing duplication among health care providers. This streamlining is a challenge, as nurses attempt to focus on outcomes of care rather than lengthy written descriptions of care (a balancing act).

THE HEALTH RECORD

The health record, or medical record, is one of the documents in which nurses must write. The health record is a documented account of a person's health, illness, or treatment in a hard copy or electronic form. Its purpose is to provide effective communication to the health care team, provide for a person's continuity of care; enable the evaluation of a person's process and health outcome; and retain its integrity over time.[5]

The above statement shows how important the health record is as a tool of communication for all health professionals involved with a patient's care. It also highlights the importance of the health record as a means of evaluating the care provided to the patient, not just for management purposes, but also for legal purposes. For this reason, the legal requirements in their documentation of which nurses must be aware will be briefly examined.

Legal principles of documentation

The following are principles of legally correct documentation, which aim to guide nurses in terms of documentation requirements.[6, 7]

Principle 1: Only document 'fact'. This means entries must be objective, with no assumptions made, with no general discussion entered and no emotive language. If opinions are stated, it should be made clear whose opinions they are.

Principle 2: Document all relevant information. Document if there is any change in a patient's condition and action taken to address that change and who was notified of the change. Document if an ordered treatment or procedure was not used and the reasons why.
Principle 3. Make contemporaneous notes. Make entries in a patient's notes as soon as possible after an event occurs with date and time clearly marked. Contemporaneous notes have greater weight as evidence than notes made at a time further from the event.
Principle 4. Records should be legible, in ink, signed, dated, and unaltered. Never obliterate a mistake or wrong entry. Leave mistakes or errors legible, draw a line through and initial them.

Other advice is to:

- ensure the patient's name and identification number is on every sheet in the health record
- read the health record, particularly the previous nursing entry before making an entry
- leave no space between entries and no space between entry and signature
- use only endorsed abbreviations, and
- do not make notes on scraps of paper for rewriting into the health record later.[8]

Minimum requirements

There are a number of minimum requirements relating to the identification and entry into a patient's **health care record**.[9]

- Records should be clearly identified as relating to a particular person.
- Each entry should be signed, with name and designation clearly identifiable.
- Orientation to the facility should include information on documentation guidelines.
- Entries should be made in a non-erasable way.
- The year, date, and time should appear on each entry. When the entry is made after an 'event', the time of the event should be noted.
- All errors should remain readable, with a line drawn through them and initialled.
- Documentation should occur sequentially, with no space between each entry.
- Only endorsed abbreviations should be used.
- Access to records should be provided only to legitimate authorised persons after proof of identification.
- The frequency of entry should be in line with the policy of the facility.

Each health care facility develops its own policies for documentation, therefore nurses must be made aware of these policies and apply them. The way in which nurses write in the health record will depend very much on the system in place in the particular setting. A number of different models exist. Traditionally, nurses have used a narrative style of documentation, lacking structure or generally only documenting medical treatment, rather than nursing care.[10] A more recent approach is the use of structured systems, based on a problem-solving approach.[11] These are:

- the Subjective, Objective, Assessment, Plan, Intervention, Evaluation, and Revision method (SOAPIER) or SOAP for short
- the Problem, Intervention, and Evaluation method (PIE), and the
- Data, Action, and Results method.

All of the above methods of structured entry into the health record are based on the problem-solving approach of the nursing process. They require concise and reflective documentation and allow nurses and others involved in patient care to see progress towards the patient care goals.

Because of time constraints on nurses, other methods of documentation in the health record are becoming more common. Documenting by 'exception' or 'variation', where only changes from the expected progress are documented, is becoming more widely used. This saves time with what may be considered unnecessary and duplicative information. This method requires the integrative approach of using the patient care plans (usually in the form of flow sheets or '**critical pathways**'). Critical pathways are defined as multidisciplinary, patient care tools, based on specific conditions. They identify core or essential components of care as well as day-to-day patient requirements that will move the patient towards discharge in a timely and consistent way.[12] The whole health care team uses the pathway to guide treatment and care and only variations from the 'norm' are documented, or charted. All positive or negative variations from the established base-lines are documented. The most attractive features of the critical pathways method of documentation are the focus on the multidisciplinary approach to care, reduction of duplication, and time saving. However, they rely on careful and regular review or evaluation.

There is criticism of the use of standardised pathways and flow sheets. It is suggested that the use of these stifle the nurse's real voice by not allowing evidence of the richness of nursing practice. They may distort views regarding patient dependency, staffing levels, and workloads and prevent a reflective type of nursing care planning.[13] Ideally, a balance should take place between lean, standardised documentation and rich, reflective nursing care documentation. However, under the current climate of budgetary restraint and focus on outcomes rather than process, the use of tick boxes, flow sheets and documentation by exception will most likely flourish. Regardless of the system of documentation, it should allow nurses (and other providers) to clearly see what care is planned for the patient and what has been given. This is of great importance for the effective and continuing care of patients in all care settings.

Looking to the future

The future of documentation involving nurses and other health care providers will involve even more standardisation and streamlining. This will allow the easy flow of information across organisation boundaries, via automated systems. More and more data will be entered directly into computerised systems, including patient observations and progress notes. Nursing care plan information will also become part of this integrated system.

Automated systems are being trialed in many and varied institutions and organisations. In some cases,[14] it is more time consuming than manual documentation as problems are ironed out, but eventually these systems should provide what is intended; that is, an efficient and effective method of communicating nursing and other health care information.

With the complexity of the health care system and the likelihood of patients to be cared for by a number of providers in different settings, a Standardised Electronic Health Record (SER) is one of the goals of the New South Wales Government.[15] The use of the SER would allow all providers to access information regarding patients and therefore ensure better continuity of care, as well as reducing duplication. There are obvious issues involving confidentiality and privacy involved in this type of system, but the New South Wales government's goal is to have it implemented within the next five years and at federal level by 2010.

The ultimate goal for the better integration of services is the patient-held electronic health record. Already, community agencies such as the Royal District Nursing Service in Victoria and other home nursing services leave the patient record in the patient's home. This ensures each nurse caring for the patient has the care plan and other information at hand. It also allows other providers of care to access this information and contribute to the record. The electronic patient-held record allows patients to take their record to health providers, who will then see a complete picture of care and care plans. Of course this system will require a large amount of infrastructure and education to ensure compatible systems and standardised language and coding.

In summary, documentation procedures and systems are evolving. They are moving from a system based on a narrative but information-rich style, to a lean, standardised, streamlined, and multidisciplinary system. The challenge for nurses is to demonstrate the richness of their practice, while communicating in a way that allows the smooth and complete flow of information in an efficient manner.

HANDOVER

Nurses need quality information at the beginning of each shift to inform them of patient care and ward activities to ensure care is maintained and continued. This information is passed on during a period called '**handover**'.[16, 17] It is most commonly a verbal communication of a patient's health status, needs, treatments, outcomes, and responses to ensure continuity of care.[18] However, with changes in work practices, the use of non-verbal handover is being trialed and increasingly used.[19]

Handover may take place in a number of forms, depending on how care is managed. The most widely used practices are: the traditional narrative handover; the bedside handover; the taped handover; and the non-verbal or written handover. Regardless of the method used, the handover should be well planned and include a number of common elements based upon the patient care plan and other documentation.[20, 21, 22, 23] The information in the handover should be patient-centred rather than a report of the nurse's own activities over the shift. Information should include:

1. background data and reason for care
2. primary medical and nursing diagnoses
3. current priority problems
4. changes in treatments or condition
5. interventions or treatments of priority problems
6. outcomes and responses to interventions or treatments
7. new orders or interventions not yet documented
8. social/emotional issues.
9. progress towards discharge.[24]

The handover may be tailored for the oncoming nurse. Therefore, when possible, it is important that the nurse performing the handover be informed of who the oncoming nurse is. A brief handover may be required for a nurse who has looked after the same patients for a number of days, where a more comprehensive handover may be required for an agency or casual nurse unfamiliar with the facility.

The traditional narrative handover

The traditional, narrative handover has been discussed widely in the nursing literature.[25, 26, 27] It has evolved from the Charge Nurse (Nurse Unit Manager) giving a verbal report on each patient in the ward and then delegating tasks to the oncoming staff. More recently it has involved each outgoing nurse providing information about the patients they have cared for to all oncoming staff. This type of handover usually takes place in a meeting room, away from the patients. It may serve a number of other functions, such as debriefing, social interaction, and training. It allows questions and provides a forum for problem-solving.

A negative aspect of the traditional verbal handover is the amount of time it takes, and having double staff on duty, yet even less than full staff on the ward. It has also been criticised for encouraging subjective, judgmental, and stereotypical attitudes among nurses,[28, 29] while the information is likely to lack planning and consistency.

The traditional handover has come under increasing scrutiny particularly in relation to nursing costs, movement towards breaking down traditional professional boundaries, and changing work practices.[30] A number of factors have come into play, which may make the traditional handover inappropriate. They include: the reduction of shift overlap times; the increased use of casual staff; and the use of shorter shifts for some staff. Therefore, alternative methods of handover are being used more widely to accommodate these changes.

The bedside handover

Bedside handovers are seen by some as the model for hospital nursing in the future, particularly as they place the patient firmly in the centre of all care activity.[31, 32] The departing nurse hands over each patient one by one to the oncoming nurse. Unlike other forms of handover, the patient has the opportunity to participate in care planning. The nursing report must be objective and carefully delivered, based on documentation in the nursing care plans and health record.

An important aspect of the bedside handover, which is not available in a taped or written handover, is the opportunity for the oncoming nurse to ask questions as well as be involved in problem-solving at the time. The patient becomes an integral part of the process and is likely to be involved with the problem-solving approach as well.

The bedside handover also provides an opportunity for other staff such as medical and allied health staff to be more involved in the plan of care for the patient. In specialised areas such as intensive care units medical staff often share in the nursing bedside handovers at the beginning of the day. Conversely, nurses are being encouraged to take more of an active role in medical ward rounds to increase collaboration, breaking down communication barriers.[33] The bedside handover provides an open forum for interdisciplinary collaboration and greater patient involvement. Involving all providers in regular handovers or reports will improve the links between them and ensure continuity of care.

The possible disadvantages of the bedside handover are few, but a major concern nurses tend to have is with confidentiality.[34, 35] Nurses are also concerned with details that may be upsetting to patients and their families, especially in such areas as oncology and palliative care.[36] In these situations a full handover at the bedside may not be appropriate. Bedside handovers may be used in combination with a closed handover away from patients.

Taped handovers

Tape recorded handovers allow nurses of the previous shift to record handover information at a time that suits them, in terms of their patient care. The recording is then played back to the oncoming shift without the need for the previous shift's presence.[37] It is argued that with the use of a systematic and structured format, the tape recorded handover ensures objective and consistent information about each patient, which is backed up by the documentation.[38]

The advantages of a tape recorded handover are:

- Nurses can record their report at a time that suits them.
- Nurses already on duty can continue to care for their patients while the oncoming nurses listen to handover.
- It can save up to 50 per cent of the time required for the traditional handover.
- The tape can be repeated to allow for flexible shift start times.
- The information is consistent in format and quality.
- It may be used to provide an update for ward doctors.
- The information can be updated if required.

The disadvantages are:

- There may be a lack of opportunity to ask questions, leading the nurse providing care with incomplete information (may be dangerous).
- The recorded information may be unclear, that is, difficult to understand for a number of reasons, which may include poor recording technique or accents that are difficult to understand.[39]

Taped handovers rely on excellent documentation. The oncoming nurse is likely to need to review the health record and care plan for clarification and guidance. Patient care may be put at risk if the documentation is incomplete. It is essential that the quality of the tape recording is good. It should therefore be checked during each recording. Clear speech is also essential. One frightening account of a poor-quality recording involved an agency nurse working in a private hospital on night duty: *'When I came on to the ward, most of the evening staff had left. I was given a tape recorder to listen to and could hardly make out what the nurse was saying. I didn't know any of the patients and was unfamiliar with the ward. It was a nightmare. The other night duty staff were not interested in helping me, as they were too busy. They were annoyed by my questions.'*

This example illustrates a problem with poor-quality recording and unclear enunciation, as well as the inappropriate use of tape recorded handover in the situation of a staff member unfamiliar with the ward. It also highlights another problem that is often encountered by casual or agency staff: the reluctance of regular staff to spend time orientating and answering questions of the casual staff. This is a very important communication issue, which needs to be tackled at management level. Part of the problem is the shorter hours worked by casual staff, and those hours are usually the busiest hours on a ward. In effect, the casual nurse is 'thrown in at the deep end'.

With the right equipment, training, backing documentation, and focus on the needs of oncoming staff, the taped handover can be a successful and efficient way of communicating.

Non-verbal handovers

Verbal handovers have been criticised as a 'form of safety net nursing' because they often include important but undocumented information (part of the oral tradition of nursing).[40] Nurses, then, rely on the verbal transfer of this information, which is often unreliable. The verbal handover is also criticised for focusing on the care already given, rather than the care required.

The non-verbal or written handover is becoming more widely used for the same reasons as taped handovers. Ideally, it involves oncoming nurses spending time reading patient and ward information prior to commencing care for their patients. Information includes: patient biographical details and information sheets; the patient care plans; ward diaries for admissions, discharges, appointments, and the most recent entries in the patient record. It also relies on nurses documenting all nurse-to-nurse communication.[41]

The use of written handovers relies heavily on excellent ward coordination (with a focus on team nursing) and of course excellent documentation. Written handovers have similar negative aspects as tape-recorded handovers. These relate to the lack of face-to-face interaction between the leaving and oncoming staff.

How to ensure consistent and high-quality handovers

Many factors ensure consistent and high-quality handovers, regardless of the mode of delivery.[42] Management factors include written guidelines for handover and the production of a standardised handover or patient information sheet for note taking. Both of these will provide format and focus for both the departing and oncoming nurse. Individual staff should pay attention to the following factors:

1. Planning: information should be consistently structured in line with guidelines, based on care plans and other documentation.
2. Timing: the verbal delivery or recording of the handover should be acceptable and appropriate for those involved. The information should be as contemporaneous as possible.
3. Setting: except for bedside handovers, the environment should be without distraction.

It is important to evaluate the handover process. Nurses should ask themselves the following questions:

- Is this the best way we can do this?
- Are we giving the information required?
- Are we duplicating anything?
- Is this the most efficient use of our time? [43]

In summary, the handover process has come under scrutiny, as the focus and pressures of the health system have changed. It is no longer adequate for nurses to rely on *ad hoc* methods, entrenched in the traditions of the past, to communicate the ongoing needs and plans for patients. Handover is a time to share information in an efficient manner, ensuring it is based on the patient care plans and other documentation. Important information must be documented and available for the oncoming nurse.

Each health setting is different even within one institution, therefore handover practices should be tailored for each specific area. A combination of handover practices may even be required in a particular area at different times over a 24-hour period. Important features that are part of the traditional narrative handover should not be forgotten. Communication involving problem-solving, debriefing and teaching should still take place as they are important not only for safe and continuing patient care but also for staff morale.

REFERRAL

Handover is the transfer of patient care within teams. Referral is another form of handover. It is the transfer of patient care from one team to another. The referral of patients from one provider to another is often essential in terms of continuity and appropriateness of care. This is particularly important as patients with diverse needs move quickly from one care setting to another.[44] Shorter lengths of hospital stay, complex, chronic conditions, and an ageing population have increased the need for referral.

The referral process is defined as a systematic, problem-solving approach helping patients utilise resources to resolve needs. It comprises a number of steps:[45]

1 establish a working relationship with the patient based on open and honest communication;
2 establish the need for referral by involving the patient in the identification of needs and possible referral alternatives;
3 set objectives for the referral by matching patient needs with realistic options;
4 explore resource availability;
5 make the referral to the resource by following the resource's protocols, remembering to share any unique patient circumstances; and

6 evaluate and follow-up the referral, to ensure the patient's expectations are met and to identify any problems that can be avoided with other referrals.

The most important communication skill the nurse can possess, in regard to referrals, is listening. A good listener will identify a need for referral. Patients may not be clear about their needs, or may not feel comfortable expressing them. A nurse with good listening skills and the ability to develop an open and trusting relationship will enable patients to express their needs. Without listening to a patient and the patient's family and friends, the need for referral may go unrecognised.

The importance of nurses' responsibility in the referral process is recognised in the guidelines of the Nurses' Association. Nurses work in varied settings, within hospitals, community, and tertiary care areas. All nurses should be aware of their responsibilities regarding referrals, regardless of whether they are formal (written) or informal (word of mouth). The following guidelines (supplied by the New South Wales Nurses' Association) apply to referrals made by registered nurses:[46]

1. Referrals should be made in consultation with the person involved.
2. The need for further assessment, likely management and treatment options should be explained.
3. The person should be advised, objectively, of services available, and therefore make an informed decision.
4. A letter of referral should be sent or accompany the person.
5. A copy of the letter should be kept with the health record.
6. If the person declines the referral, this should be documented in the health record.
7. Where the referral is of a medical nature, the person should be referred back to their regular medical practitioner.
8. Where the person does not have a regular doctor, they should be encouraged to make contact with one.
9. The person may be directly referred to a public hospital outpatient clinic.
10. Where practicable, the person should be contacted following referral, to discuss the outcome and satisfaction with the referral.
11. If attempts to contact the person are unsuccessful, then this should be documented in the health record.
12. If, on contact with the person, it is revealed that the person did not action the referral, then the nurse should be encouraging to do so. If the person fails to act on the referral, local protocols should be followed (e.g. notify senior management) and record this in the health record.

These guidelines highlight the importance of documentation in the communication process of referrals.

Communication between providers in the health care system is sometimes inefficient and often inadequate, particularly between referring and receiving agencies.[47] Referral is a two-way form of communication. It is a communication process, involving sending information, receiving information, decoding information, and feeding back information.[48] There is a relationship between the referring agency or individual and the receiving agency or individual. For successful and appropriate referrals, both need to be actively involved with the process. Institutional and personal barriers prevent the smooth flow of information. Referral information passes through 'filters', and the more filters it passes through, the greater chance it will be changed, untimely, or even lost. The fewer filters information must pass through, the more likely the information is to be transferred and correctly received (just like 'Chinese whispers'). Referral is a process, relying on both organisational and personal systems for success.

Nurses are the only health care providers in the hospital system working with all patients. They are therefore in the ideal position to begin the referral process, which is the recognition that there is a need. They may not be required to follow the rest of the process through, but the recognition of the need is the most important step.

Referral systems: breaking down walls/building bridges

As mentioned, there are a number of organisational and personal barriers that hamper effective referrals. These are set out in brief.

Organisational barriers to effective referrals include:

- conflicts over control of patient information
- unclear priorities for staff
- unclear roles and responsibilities
- high staff turnover
- poor documentation in health records
- continuity of care not seen as important priority, and
- lack of technical systems for information transfer (computers, fax, and email).

Personal barriers to effective referrals include a lack of:

- collaboration skills
- knowledge about roles of other agencies
- problem-solving skills
- coordination skills
- prioritising skills, and
- accountability.

Personal approaches

Most of the personal skills required for effective referral can be addressed with education and support. For instance, collaboration skills can be promoted by senior staff and educators. Nurses must break down interprofessional barriers by learning to collaborate with others involved in patient care. Failure to collaborate is not usually due to ill intent but a lack of collaboration skills.[49] Basic communication skills include using an attentive style of communication and being willing to articulate one's viewpoint, having a 'give and take' relationship, caring, trusting, and respecting one another. It is also important that nurses accept their own power and the power of others appropriately, as failure to do so has been shown to block collaboration.[50] In the past nurses may have been resentful towards other health professionals performing roles which were once the sole province of nurses. Professional boundaries are now blurred in many health settings, so nurses should be confident and comfortable with their own roles, to ensure continuing care of their patients. Collaboration is essential.

The use of critical pathways, or other forms of care plans which focus on the continuum of care, help with using a multidisciplinary approach as well as looking beyond an acute phase of health care. Education and the support of protocols and guidelines for referrals also help staff to identify needs and follow through with the process.

The roles and responsibilities of staff in relation to patient referral must be clear. For example, they should be well aware if there is a 'discharge planner' who will coordinate all aspects of referral, and how to access the discharge planner. Nurses should understand the roles of others involved in their patients' care such as social workers and occupational therapists. This will prevent duplication while ensuring that the continuing needs of patients are met. One of the major problems with unsuccessful discharge planning is the lack of awareness of or ambiguity of roles.[51]

Nurses may not be aware of the priority they should give to the identification of referral needs and the subsequent referral process. This could be addressed by education, but should also be supported in the patient care plan. For instance, an awareness that discharge planning should start on admission is vital and written discharge plans should be incorporated in the care plans.

The use of a screening tool or flow chart for the identification and subsequent referral actions help nurses and other providers to ensure referrals are made appropriately and efficiently, in time for the discharge or further treatment.[52] Such tools provide a more reliable system, in an attempt to prevent patients 'slipping through the net' and being discharged from hospital without the support services they require.

In essence, nurses need to talk with others involved in ongoing patient care. Direct communication will help in the development of a good working relationship and the breaking down of personal barriers. Although it might seem terribly old fashioned, a face to a name or a voice over the phone will help a relationship for the future. It is often a good idea to invite the people to whom patients are referred to come and speak about what they do and how best to approach them.

Organisational approaches

The removal of personal barriers to effective referrals can only be achieved with the support of the organisation. Systems must be in place that allow timely and smooth flow of information from one setting to another, or from one provider to another. This begins with organisational or area protocols and guidelines for referrals. These guidelines should address roles and responsibilities to ensure there is no ambiguity or confusion.

The organisational model chosen for the management of continuing care for patients will also determine the success of referrals. For instance, there are a number of alternatives available: the primary nurse system; the discharge planner; the liaison nurse; general bedside staff; and a multiprofessional collaboration model based on case management.

It is suggested that the primary nurse model works well in specialist areas,[53] whereas the use of general bedside staff as discharge planners tends not to work well unless they are clear about their own role and accountability in regard to discharge planning. With the increased use of casual staff common in non-specialist areas, the use of general bedside staff as discharge planners is not recommended. Most successful models for coordination of referrals, and therefore discharge planning, are the use of a discharge planner whose sole responsibility is planning discharges. However, this relies on the adequate availability of the discharge planner and the early recognition for the need of such a service by the staff nurses. A case management model that involves more than one professional is also widely and successfully used.

The liaison nurse is a nurse from a community-based nursing organisation, based in the acute sector. The liaison nurse acts as a discharge planner by identifying potential patients and ensuring they are adequately prepared for transfer to the particular community-based care. Many hospitals find the liaison nurse provides an excellent link with the community and may also provide essential education and support to staff. In effect, the liaison nurse provides a system with little filter. The liaison nurse can also provide feedback to nurses after the patient has been discharged.

To overcome problems with interorganisational communication and referrals, many large hospitals are developing their own post discharge or post acute care services. This makes the transition from hospital to home more seamless. However, it still relies on patients being referred to the service.

In summary, the roles and responsibilities of discharge planning (as an example of referring) within an organisation must be well thought out in terms of the types of patients, nursing workforce issues, area specialties and links and availability of community resources.

Information transfer is facilitated when referral data passes through fewer filters.[54] Currently, many hospitals are attempting to improve their communication systems by reducing the number of filters through which information passes. For example, a number of hospitals in New South Wales are using DOCFACS, which is an automatically generated, faxed discharge summary principally for general practitioners. The topic of referral from general practitioners to tertiary or specialist services, and information provided back on discharge, is covered in detail in Chapter 11 by Max Kamien.

Nursing services are also developing computer-generated referral systems from databases maintained by nurses and allied health staff. The Post Acute Care Service based at the Prince of Wales Hospital is trialling one such system. These systems rely on well-structured and complete documentation in the health record.

Forging closer links between acute and community services are essential for appropriate and effective referrals. A number of strategies are effective for improving links. For example, a community nursing service such as the Royal District Nursing Service (RDNS) in Victoria works closely with 'Hospital in the Home' and post acute programs in various hospitals as a provider of nursing services. They orientate hospital staff by taking them 'on the road' for a couple of days; they have regular meetings with hospital staff; are involved with joint staff education sessions; and communicate daily with case managers by phone. Secondment is another strategy being employed to improve links between community and acute services. This is a strategy currently in use by the Post Acute Care Facilitation Unit (PACFU) of the North Western Health Care network in Victoria.[55] It is found that professional exchanges or secondments from hospitals and community service providers result in better understanding of the post acute program and therefore more appropriate and timely referrals to it.

Follow-up procedures are a vital element of the referral system. An organisation that makes referrals needs to evaluate the outcomes of the referrals. The only way they can do this is by receiving information from the agency or individuals to whom they referred. Most acute care service based nurses are involved in some part of the referral process, even if it is only the identification of the need for referral. However, they may be unaware of the outcomes and consequences of their referrals or discharge plans.

Carefully designed feedback processes from services receiving referrals should result in a positive impact on care planning from the referral source. An example of a feedback process used by the PACFU is as follows:

- individualised feedback is given to referring practitioners, informing them of the outcomes of the care plans they devised
- participation in data collection activities with community services and the feedback of this information to the discharging hospitals

- regular reports to ward staff containing aggregated data on referral rates, the accuracy, timeliness, completeness, and appropriateness of referrals, and
- participating in hospital and community committees relating to patients' continuum of care.

Improving links and breaking down barriers can be achieved geographically. Integrated Care Centres are being developed, where multiple services are located under one roof. Services may include: community health nursing, mental health care, and some acute care services. The purpose of these centres is to provide an environment where services are coordinated, thereby avoiding duplication. However, they still rely on a collaborative approach by all staff for this to happen. If there is a 'power struggle' between agencies, the system will fail.

The successful transfer of information will depend on the type of information involved. It is argued that more specific, concise information will be conveyed successfully, rather than more general, ambiguous, or interpretive information (lean versus rich).[56] The use of standardised forms and even standardised language such as nursing codes will improve the transfer of data from one organisation to another.

Information technology provides nurses and other health professionals involved in referrals with a great opportunity to transfer information effectively and efficiently. The provision of fax machines and the use of email ensures the timely transfer of information. The availability of mobile phones makes community services staff more accessible to hospital staff.

Looking to the future, more and more computer-generated information will be used to coordinate care from one service to another. The New South Wales Health Council states that information technology will become a core feature of responsive service delivery and recommends the following changes:

- the development of an Electronic Health Record for every individual in New South Wales;
- improvement of links between patient information systems within hospitals, between hospitals, and community health teams and between hospitals and general practitioners; and
- the establishment of a Unique Patient Identifier for every individual in New South Wales, so care providers can identify with certainty the patient they are dealing with, regardless of where the patient has entered the health system.[57]

The development of a computerised, comprehensive referral system should:

- provide patients and providers instant access to information on a range of health care and community services;
- streamline interagency referrals and intake procedures;
- capture patient service utilisation history across multiple providers; and
- reduce the need for patients to repeat the same information to different providers.[58]

In an attempt to better link community services and set up systems for seamless care, systems such as the Community Based Health Information System (CBHIS) are being set up with a strong referral infrastructure. The CBHIS will be used in at least four states of Australia.

Other services attempt to link care providers to improve communication and reduce duplication of services and research such as the Victorian Centre for Ambulatory Care Innovation. One of the Centre's aims is to foster ambulatory care models based on a multidisciplinary care team approach, which are coordinated, cooperative, longitudinal, and integrated.[59] This collaborative approach could be seen as the aim of health care in any setting.

In summary, patient referral is an essential aspect of communication in relation to continuity of care. The changes in the way our health system operates have increased the pressure on nurses to ensure continuity of care. Decreasing length of hospital stay, the fragmentation of services and the likelihood of a patient requiring a number of different health and community services for one particular illness or incident have placed a greater emphasis on the effective transfer of patient information. The process of referral must be supported by organisational systems that allow the smooth and uninterrupted transfer of information. The roles and responsibilities of nurses should be clearly defined in relation to referring. Nurses are required to use effective personal communication skills to build bridges and break down barriers between themselves and other providers of care, both within their own setting and between organisations.

CONCLUSION

In many ways, nursing is all about communication with patients and with other care providers. Nurses' roles and responsibilities are many and varied. At the core of what nurses do is taking care of patients, ensuring they receive not only the clinical care they require, but also other aspects of care such as emotional and social care. To provide this care and ensure a continuation of care, nurses require a vision looking beyond the immediate needs of the patient. Both the handover and referral processes address this continuation of care and both require insight, planning, and delivery. Supportive documentation is the link in the chain and nurses are required to strike a balance between rich but time-consuming narrative documentation and lean but efficient documentation. The traditions of the past are giving way to the changes of today and the future and the way in which nurses communicate with each other and other health care providers. These changes should place the patient firmly in the centre of all communication.

NOTES

The author would like to acknowledge the assistance of Fiona McCormack, Centre Manager, Royal District Nursing Service, Victoria; Neville Board, NSW Department of Health; and Toby Mathieson, NSW Department of Health.

1 Anderson, M.A. and Helms, L.B. Talking about patients: communication and continuity of care. *Journal of Cardiovascular Nursing* 2000, vol. 14, no. 3, pp. 15–28.

2 Department of Human Services, Victoria. *Effective Discharge Strategy. Background Paper: A Framework for Effective Discharge.* December 1998.

3 Page, C. Looking to the Future: Critical Pathways, in J. Richmond (ed.), *Nursing Documentation: Writing What We Do.* Ausmed Publications, Melbourne, 1997, pp. 87–99.

4 Moorhouse, C. Is written documentation essential to good nursing practice? *Nursing Documentation: A Symposium to Address Emerging Concerns.* Papers from the symposium held at the Royal Women's Hospital, Melbourne, 22 September 1995.

5 New South Wales Health Department. *Principles for Creation, Management, Storage and Disposal of Health Care Records.* Circular No. 98/59, 1998.

6 Taylor, K. Legal issues for nurses: defensive nursing practice, Lamp 1997, vol. 54, no. 4, pp. 12–13.

7 Jamieson, A. Legal Issues in Documentation, in J. Richmond (ed.), *Nursing Documentation: Writing What We Do.* Ausmed Publications, Melbourne, 1997, pp. 63–9.

8 New South Wales Health Department. *Principles for Creation, Management, Storage and Disposal of Health Care Records.* Circular No. 98/59, 1998.

9 New South Wales Health Department. *Principles for Creation, Management, Storage and Disposal of Health Care Records.* Circular No. 98/59, 1998.

10 Schulz-Robinson, S. 'A political imperative: make nurses' work visible by documentation', in J. Richmond (ed.), *Nursing Documentation: Writing What We Do.* Ausmed Publications, Melbourne, 1997, pp. 173–9.

11 Eggland, E. and Heineman, D. *Nursing Documentation: Charting, Recording and Reporting.* J.B. Lippincott Company, Philadelphia, 1994, pp. 119–21.

12 Page, C. Looking to the future: critical pathways, in J. Richmond (ed.), *Nursing Documentation: Writing What We Do.* Ausmed Publications, Melbourne, 1997, pp. 87–99.

13 Schulz-Robinson, S. *A Political Imperative: make nurses' work visible by documentation,* in J. Richmond (ed.), *Nursing Documentation: Writing What We Do*, pp. 173–9.

14 Allan, J. and Englebright, J. Patient centred documentation: an efficient use of clinical information systems, *Journal of Nursing Administration,* 2000, vol. 30, no. 2, pp. 90–5.

15 New South Wales Government. *Report of the New South Wales Health Council—A Better Health System for New South Wales,* Sydney, 2000.

16 Miller, C. Ensuring continuing care: styles and efficiency of the handover process, *Australian Journal of Advanced Nursing,* 1998, vol .16 no. 1, pp. 23–7.

17 Prouse, M. A study of the use of tape recorded handovers. *Nursing Times,* 1995, vol. 91 no. 49, pp. 40–1.
18 Eggland, E. and Heinemann D. *Nursing Documentation: Charting, Recording and Reporting.* J.B. Lippincott Company, Philadelphia, 1994, pp. 119–21.
19 Kennedy, J. An evaluation of non verbal handover, *Professional Nurse,* 1999, vol. 14, no. 6, pp. 391–4.
20 Eggland, E. and Heinemann, D. *Nursing Documentation: Charting, Recording and Reporting.* J.B. Lippincott Company, Philadelphia, 1994, pp. 119–21.
21 Miller, C. Ensuring continuing care: styles and efficiency of the handover process, *Australian Journal of Advanced Nursing,* 1999, vol. 16, no. 8, pp. 23–7.
22 Prouse, M. A study of the use of tape recorded handovers, *Nursing Times,* 1995, vol. 91, no. 49, pp. 40–1.
23 Webster, J. Practitioner-centred research: an evaluation of the implementation of the bedside hand-over, *Journal of Advanced Nursing,* 1999, vol. 30, no. 6, pp. 1375–82.
24 McKenna, L. Improving the nursing handover report. *Professional Nurse,* 1997, vol. 12 no. 9: pp. 637–9.
25 Parker, J., Gardner, G. and Wiltshire, J. Handover: the collective narrative of nursing practice, *The Australian Journal of Advanced Nursing,* 1992, vol. 9 no. 3, pp. 31–7.
26 Parker, J. Handovers in a changing health care climate, *Australian Nursing Journal,* 1996, vol. 4, no. 5, pp. 22–6.
27 Miller, C. Ensuring continuing care: styles and efficiency of the handover process, *Australian Journal of Advanced Nursing,* 1998, vol. 16, no. 1, pp. 23–7.
28 Kennedy, J. An evaluation of non verbal handover, *Professional Nurse,* 1998, vol. 14 no. 1, pp. 391–4.
29 McKenna, L. Improving the nursing handover report, *Professional Nurse,* 1997, vol. 12, no. 9, pp. 637–9.
30 Parker, J. Handovers in a changing health care climate, *Australian Nursing Journal,* 1996, vol. 4, no. 5, pp. 22–6.
31 Parker, J. Handovers in a changing health care climate, *Australian Nursing Journal,* 1996, vol. 4, no. 5, pp. 22–6.
32 Webster, J. Practitioner–centred research: an evaluation of the implementation of the bedside hand-over, *Journal of Advanced Nursing,* 1999, vol. 30, no. 6, pp. 1375–82.
33 Wright, S., Bowkett, J. and Bray, K. The communication gap in the ICU—a possible solution, *Nursing in Critical Care,* 1996, vol. 1, no. 5, pp. 241–4.
34 Parker, J. Handovers in a changing health care climate, *Australian Nursing Journal,* 1996, vol. 4, no. 5, pp. 22–6.
35 Miller, C. Ensuring continuing care: styles and efficiency of the handover process, *Australian Journal of Advanced Nursing,* 1998, vol. 16, no. 1, pp. 23–7.
36 McKenna, L. and Walsh, K. Changing handover practices: one private hospital's experiences, *International Journal of Nursing Practice,* 1997, vol. 3, pp. 128–32.
37 Miller, C. Ensuring continuing care: styles and efficiency of the handover process, *Australian Journal of Advanced Nursing,* 1998, vol. 16, no. 1, pp. 23–7.

38 Prouse, M. A study of the use of tape recorded handovers, *Nursing Times,* 1995, vol. 91, no. 49, pp. 40–1.

39 Miller, C. Ensuring continuing care: styles and efficiency of the handover process, *Australian Journal of Advanced Nursing,* 1998, vol. 16, no. 1, pp. 23–7.

40 Kennedy, J. An evaluation of non verbal handover, *Professional Nurse,* 1998, vol. 14, no. 1, pp. 391–4.

41 Kennedy, J. An evaluation of non verbal handover, *Professional Nurse,* 1998, vol. 14, no. 1, pp. 391–4.

42 Miller, C. Ensuring continuing care: styles and efficiency of the handover process, *Australian Journal of Advanced Nursing,* 1998, vol. 16, no. 1, pp. 23–7.

43 Miller, C. Ensuring continuing care: styles and efficiency of the handover process, *Australian Journal of Advanced Nursing,* 1998, vol. 16, no. 1, pp. 23–7.

44 McGuire, S., Gerber, D. and Clemen-Stone, S. Meeting the diverse needs of clients in the community: effective use of the referral process. *Nursing Outlook,* 1996, vol. 44, no. 5, pp. 218–22.

45 McGuire, S., Gerber, D. and Clemen-Stone, S. Meeting the diverse needs of clients in the community: effective use of the referral process. *Nursing Outlook,* 1996, vol. 44, no. 5, pp. 218–22.

46 Illiffe, J. Professional team: referral responsibilities, *Lamp,* 1997, vol. 54 no. 1, p. 19.

47 Anderson, M.A. and Helms, L.B. Extended care referral after hospital discharge, *Research in Nursing and Health,* 1998, vol. 21, pp. 385–94.

48 Anderson, M.A. and Helms, L.B. Extended care referral after hospital discharge, *Research in Nursing and Health,* 1998, vol. 21, pp. 385–94.

49 Van Ess Coeling, H., Cukr, L. Communication styles that promote perceptions of collaboration, quality and nurse satisfaction, *Journal of Nursing Care Quality,* 2000, vol. 14, no. 2, pp. 63–74.

50 Van Ess Coeling, H., Cukr, L. Communication styles that promote perceptions of collaboration, quality and nurse satisfaction, pp. 63–74.

51 Grimmer, K., Hedges, G. and Moss, J. Staff perceptions of discharge planning: a challenge for quality improvement, *Australian Health Review,* 1999, vol. 22, no. 3, pp. 95–109.

52 McGinley, S., Baus, E., Gyza, K., Johnson, K., Lipton, S., Magee, M., Moore, F. and Wojtyak, D. Multidisciplinary discharge planning: developing a process, *Nursing Management,* 1996, vol. 27, no. 10, pp. 55–60.

53 Anderson, M.A. and Helms, L. An assessment of discharge planning models: communication in referrals for home care, *Orthopaedic Nursing,* 1993, vol. 12, no. 4, pp. 41–9.

54 Anderson, M.A. and Helms, L. B. Extended care referral after hospital discharge, *Research in Nursing and Health,* 1998, vol. 21, pp. 385–94.

55 Acute Health Division, Quality Branch, Department of Health, Victoria. Post Acute Care Program. *North Western Health Care Network Care Planning Development Project.* Department of Health Services, Victoria, 2000.

56 Anderson, M.A., Helms, L.B. Talking about patients: communication and continuity of care, *Journal of Cardiovascular Nursing,* 2000, vol. 14, no. 3, pp. 15–28.

57 New South Wales Government. *Report of the New South Wales Health Council—A Better Health System for New South Wales.* Sydney, 2000.

58 Gaudet, L. Electronic referrals and data sharing: can it work for health care and social service providers? *Journal of Case Management,* 1996, vol. 5, no. 2, pp. 72–7.

59 Victorian Centre for Ambulatory Care Innovation. *Charter for Change: VCACI Mission.* Department of Health Services, Victoria, 2000.

11

Good referral letters and good replies

Max Kamien

The functioning of interdisciplinary teams is particularly dependent on good communication. In this chapter, I will focus on communications between general practitioners (**GPs**), specialists, and hospitals, since these are the most common and most complained about forms of communication. The author of this chapter is both a GP and a **specialist** physician. This chapter is written from both these perspectives. It is intended to be useful to both referers and referees.

GPs refer about 6 per cent of all patient problems to a specialist or a hospital. In most cases this results in a reply communication from a specialist or a hospital registrar to the referring general practitioner. Similar forms of communication occur between GPs and allied health professionals. Good communication facilitates rapport between health professionals and institutions. Poor or absent communication can do the opposite and on occasions can constitute a danger to a patient's (or client's) well-being.

A Medline search from January 1966 to February 2000 produced 69 communications on this topic; 37 commented on GPs' letters to specialists and hospitals; 15 on specialist or hospital letters to GPs; and 10 included an analysis of both letters to specialists and replies from them. Only one of these papers was complimentary in its findings.[1] A further 7 papers describe experiments with structured or electronic communications aimed at correcting some of the deficiencies recorded in this medical literature.

GPS' LETTERS

Chief criticisms of GPs' letters are inadequate information about the patient,[2] including neglect of psychosocial, cultural, religious, and health belief systems that could complicate management,[3] and GPs' failure to state their reasons and objectives for the referral and their expectations as a result of it.[4] Some specialists also feel that the likelihood of a correct diagnosis is reduced by lack of a detailed referral letter.[5]

REASONS FOR REFERRAL

The reason for referral is rarely for diagnosis but much more likely to be for an opinion on management or for a procedure.[6] Sometimes a referral is for the peace of mind of a patient and is asking for specialist affirmation of a life or lifestyle threatening diagnosis or management decision (e.g. epilepsy, Parkinson's disease, or refusal to recommend renewal of a driver's licence).

PUBLIC HOSPITALS

Public hospital outpatient clinics often have long waiting lists and specialists working in them are critical of GPs' referral letters that do not provide adequate information about the urgency with which an appointment needs to be made. Particular examples are breast clinics in which the GP's assessment of the likelihood or unlikelihood of a carcinoma is appreciated and has been found accurate.[7] For similar reasons, oncologists particularly want to know a patient's general medical status.[8] Other negative examples of GPs' letters reported in the medical literature were from a back clinic in which less than a third of the referring letters contained the patient's age, onset and duration of symptoms, and the results of special tests such as X-rays. In addition only 8 per cent of those letters mentioned the patient's bowel or bladder function.[9] Referral letters to obesity clinics have also been found wanting, even omitting data on body weight and height. In one Swedish study waist circumference was mentioned in only five of 500 letters, and investigations that may point towards the co-morbidity of the metabolic syndrome were present in only 7 per cent of letters.[10] In Western Australia, a senior endocrinologist with an interest in obesity wrote to doctors whose referral letter was '*too brief and contained inadequate details*'. He requested a full clinical history, details of previous treatments and their efficacy, the involvement of other specialists and their reports, and photocopies of relevant laboratory tests. He went on to explain that such information would accelerate their patient's position on the current eight-month waiting list.[11] Through administrative error, one patient received this letter and complained to her GP that his letter was unprofessional and that this was affecting her access to treatment. The GP obliged with a more informative referral.

SPECIALIST LETTERS

The main GP criticisms of **specialist letters** were that they often misinterpreted, ignored, or failed to answer the GP's questions and contained little or no educational content.[12, 13] A particular annoyance is the wasteful repeating of recent investigations that have been enclosed with the GP's referral letter.

GPs also want a diagnosis, the results of physical findings and investigations, details of treatment options, the expected side effects of treatment,[14] and whether further investigations are to be performed. In particular the referring GP wishes to know the expected outcome of the treatment, long-term prognosis and what the patient has been told.[15, 16]

Patients with life-threatening disease need a common and constant message from their medical attendants. Mixed or different opinions often lead to insecurity and the seeking of further opinions from conventional medicos and alternative practitioners. Specialists who take over the patient and fail to communicate with their GP reduce the chance for effective advocacy for the patient. One example is a third-party view of the effect of chemotherapy or other powerful medications on the patient's usual lifestyle.

Intended follow up is also important especially if it is going to involve other doctors who have been called in by the original specialist.[17] GPs, as the primary care physicians, prefer to be given the option of on-referral to other specialists or at least the opportunity for discussion. It is also helpful for GP, specialist, and patient to be clear about who is going to be responsible for changing and maintaining the patient's medication regime or designated parts of it.

None of this information is useful if it cannot be read. Handwritten hospital discharge summaries are a particular problem with 50 per cent being reported to be illegible.[18] Nevertheless, GPs prefer immediate concise legible handwritten summaries containing diagnoses, medications, and follow up, to lengthy and delayed typewritten discharge letters. After major events, such as surgery or a death, a telephone call is courteous and always appreciated.[19]

REASONS FOR MUTUAL DISSATISFACTION

Clearly there is much mutual dissatisfaction about written communication between GPs and specialists. The reasons are both technical and attitudinal. For GPs technical reasons are the lack of a good up-to-date health summary and drug sheet that can be readily photocopied and sent with a referral letter.

Attitudinal reasons relate to a poor understanding by specialists about the general practitioners' medical task and GPs' understanding of the thinking process of specialists. The ideal tasks of general practice are described in Figure 11.1.

The thinking of general practitioners is to ask what is the most likely cause and then to think about life-threatening things that they should not miss.[20] Specialists and specialists in training have chosen to be knowledgeable in a circumscribed area of medicine. They also think about the most likely cause but spend a lot more time, energy, and expense in excluding very rare possibilities. They expect GPs to act as gatekeepers to their care,[21] and to provide sufficient background information for them to readily apply their expertise.

EXCLUDE serious illness	**TREAT** common illness	**MANAGE** multiple problems
PROVIDE advocacy and continuing care	**CARE** for the dying	**PROVIDE** domiciliary care
ANTICIPATE disease	**PROMOTE** healthy lifestyle	**LOOK AFTER** aggregate human beings over time

Figure 11.1 The task of general practice

Specialists and hospital registrars also need an understanding of the conditions in which many **GP letters** are written. Urgent referrals as a result of a house call will, of necessity, contain only relatively brief details in a handwritten letter. Other reasons behind poor GP referrals result from a view that it is not worth putting effort into a referral that may be skimmed or ignored, request for a referral at the patient's insistence rather than medical need, demand for referral without consultation, and specialist request for each separate consultation or after self-referral of the patient.

These issues have ethical and potential medico-legal consequences and require further discussion.

ETHICS

Some patients demand what their GP considers to be an inappropriate referral. According to the Australian Medical Association code of ethics, this is their right.[22] Not infrequently the patient is unaware that their GP can perform the task required and when informed withdraws their request. An example is the well patient who requests a referral to a dermatologist for an annual skin cancer check. If after explanation the patient still wants the referral then it should be given. One approach is to state, in the letter to the specialist, that the reason for referral is the patient's request and that the GP is more than happy to take over the patient's continuing annual skin check up.

LAW

More difficult is the patient who self-refers to a specialist and then expects a backdated referral. The specialist's receptionist may also phone to ask for the referral. They may also ask for a new referral for each visit when the GP has previously written a referral for twelve months or longer.

The *Medicare Benefits Schedule Book* provides clear definitions on 'what is a referral and what is a single course of treatment'.[23] A GP should never allow him- or herself to be put in the position of committing any illegality against the Health Insurance Commission. One approach is to explain these issues to the patient or to the specialist's receptionist and gently finish the explanation with the question: 'Do you really want me to put my good name and medical career on the line so that you can claim a higher rebate from Medicare?'

CONTEXT AND VALUE-ADDING

Most articles in the medical literature focus on the content of letters. Few focus on the context of the consultation or on the issues of professionalism and courtesy.

The referring doctor knows the presenting history, past history, social history, and the patient's current medications. He or she does not need a reiteration of what they already know and have (or should have) included in their referral letter. What they want and need is a value-added reply. This should include a description of a consulting doctor's reasoning, especially where there are several possible management options. In future the referring doctor will increasingly want to know if this reasoning has taken into account the evidence-based literature or whether it depends only upon personal experience.

Context also includes an awareness of the consultant doctor's place in the scheme of the patient's ongoing care. This ongoing care could be likened to a medical symphony ideally conducted by the patient's personal doctor, who will have an overview of the main themes and act as the patient's advocate. At various points in that symphony, the virtuoso specialist is required to perform a cadenza, which when completed will have added to the quality of the symphony and enable it to proceed to its optimal conclusion. A failure to understand this context can, on occasion, result in tragedy for the patient when there is no clear division of responsibility for the immediate care of the patient with a severe, chronic, or rare disorder.

Professionalism from the general practitioner requires the provision of most if not all of the information laid down in the checklist in Figure 11.2. In time this will be made easier by up-to-date computerised records. A corresponding checklist for specialists and hospital registrars is produced as Figure 11.3.

Professionalism on the part of the specialist entails reading the referring letter, answering any specific questions, and replying as quickly as possible. The true professional also does not mindlessly repeat recent investigations that are

GP's details
- provider number
- period referral valid
- reason for referral
- expectation of it
- suggested responsibility for follow up
- degree of urgency

History of presenting complaint
- physical findings
- pertinent measurements e.g. height, weight, girth, growth development
- copies of investigation results
- diagnoses
- current medications
- what patient has been told

Past medical history
- details of previous treatments of current problem
- their efficacy
- involvement of other specialists

Special considerations
- health insurance status
- unusual health beliefs or religious practices
- pertinent psychosocial factors
- medico-legal concerns
- allergies

Family history
- is writing and name legible?

Figure 11.2 Checklist for GP referrals

included in or with the referring letter, but uses this information to expedite management and save money.[24]

Courtesy includes attributing credit where it is due and above all, addressing the reply to the doctor who wrote the referring letter. Hospital registrars are notorious for addressing their letters to the LMO (local medical officer), without the slightest insight into their lack of manners or the sense of alienation this produces in a referring doctor. Despite decades of articles on the topic and the new 'instant' technologies of the facsimile and e-mail, communication between the public hospital system and GPs is still described as a 'giant black hole'.[25, 26, 27]

MEDICO-LEGAL

Letters of referral and replies to them are not without legal hazard. Patients often open an envelope and read the referring letter. Uncalled for comments or attempts at alerting the specialist to psychosomatic disorder by using descriptions such as neurotic, frequent attender, or heart-sink patient may well come back to haunt the referring GP in the form of complaints to doctor review committees.[28] Care should be taken to convey sensitive information by phone

Addressed
- to referring doctor (not LMO)

Content
- brief reiteration of history
- physical findings
- diagnosis
- pertinent and further investigations

Medications
- name and dose of drug
- mode of delivery
- expected side effects
- available, affordable outside hospital?

Outcome
- prognosis
- what patient has been told
- psychosocial concerns

Follow up
- role of specialist or hospital
- involvement of other consultants in future management

Continuing medical education
- reasoning behind decisions
- whether evidence-based

Last check
- are letter and my signature legible?
- included side effects of any operation?
- have I answered all GP's questions?
- has my reply added value to the referring doctor's letter?

Figure 11.3 Checklist for specialist and hospital letters

or by asking the specialist to contact the referring doctor prior to the patient's appointment. It is in the patient's and the specialist's interests to regard such a request as a significant red flag and comply with it.

A further safeguard for doctor and patient is for the doctor to dictate the referral letter in front of the patient and then send them a copy. This should also help them to be clear about why they are seeing a specialist and what has been asked of that specialist.[29]

IMPROVING COMMUNICATION

The evidence from the medical literature is that structured, standardised referral letters are shorter but contain more useful information than narrative letters.[30] An early and useful example of a structured referral letter is part of the Royal Australian College of General Practitioners (RACGP) health record entitled 'Request for Consultation'. It has headings for much of the pertinent information already mentioned in this chapter and encourages the enclosure of health summaries and other reports. There is some evidence that a clearly legible, comprehensive health summary establishes the bona fides and apparent competence of the referring doctor, forestalls unnecessary repeat investigations and encourages a hospital to return the patient to the referring doctor.[31] A legible up-to-date health summary is also the key to shared care with GP colleagues in the same practice, either for cross-consultation or for cover when the regular GP is unavailable.

Increasing computerisation of medical records should ensure that medical software companies develop these pro formas into a truly helpful and professional format.

The same principles apply to specialist and especially hospital letters where computer-generated correspondence has been preferred by house staff and increased the likelihood of their completing a timely and better discharge summary.[32, 33] GPs have found these letters easier and quicker to interpret.[34, 35] GPs have also preferred a computer printout format, which has been easy to enter into their medical record.[36]

THREE BIRDS WITH ONE STONE?

Secretarial and medical workload and the economics of practice management will always be an impediment to producing good referral letters and good replies. This results in a particular problem for specialists and hospital registrars who often try to kill two and sometimes three birds with one stone. They try to use the one letter as their own consultation record, as a communication to the referring doctor, and increasingly as a communication to the patient.

An increasing number of doctors are following the practice of accountants, solicitors, and dentists in providing patients with a letter recapitulating, reinforcing, and summarising the main points of their consultation. Patients appreciate this service. One study showed that patients were just as satisfied to receive a copy of the letter to the GP as to receive a letter addressed directly to them.[37] Similarly, two studies have shown that a majority of GPs found that the copies of the letters to patients were 'at least as helpful, if not more so', than the type of clinic letter they usually received.[38, 39]

Perhaps the best compromise lies in writing to the referring doctor, paying particular attention to the clarity of the section on what the patient was told, and sending a copy to the patient. Of course exceptions will occur, such as the breaking or anticipating of bad news, where it could be uncaring or unethical to send a patient a copy of the letter to the general practitioner.[40] In this case, it would be necessary to write a separate letter to the doctor and the patient. A child development clinic in the United Kingdom found that information specific to the GP was required in only five of every 100 letters.[41]

VOCATIONAL TRAINING

Over the last two decades English-speaking medical schools and vocational training programs have put an increasing emphasis on the development of verbal communication skills. Written communication skills have been accorded a lower priority but are beginning to find their way into the curricula of vocational training programs.[42]

FEEDBACK

Regular review of referral letters is now part of the duties of external clinical teachers when visiting RACGP Training Program registrars in their clinical setting. Such practices also need to extend to hospital registrars.

Hospital consultants delegate discharge letters to these registrars. However, it is rare for the consultants to check even a small sample of these letters for timeliness, style, accuracy, relevance, or courtesy. Registrars do much of the work of hospitals but they are acutely aware that it is the consultant's name that is at the top of the bed and not theirs. This mutual awareness does not seem to extend to letter writing. Private specialists usually write courteous letters to the referring doctor. It would severely affect their private practice if they did not. Consultants, and the hospital administration, should ensure that those writing letters in their name keep up the same standards, especially where the anonymity of the harassed GP and harassed hospital registrar tends towards a poorer performance.[43] Audit of handwritten hospital discharge summaries, particularly their legibility and turnaround time, should be part of vocational training and ongoing quality assurance.[44, 45] A rating scale to evaluate the written communication skills of residents has already been developed.[46] The scoring methods could be easily adapted to the two checklists in this chapter.

GPs get some feedback from specialist and hospital discharge letters. They also get feedback from patients and from a knowledge of their outcome over time. Specialists rarely get feedback either good or bad. I recall reading (but unfortunately cannot find the reference) a letter from an orthopaedic surgeon who remarked that after having performed 1200 hip arthroplasties he had received his first letter from a general practitioner informing him that the operation had revolutionised the life of a patient. That sort of generous and positive feedback is appreciated and should be given more often.

Giving negative feedback is more problematic. Many GPs would feel too diffident to convey their displeasure to specialists and in those parts of the world with established and traditional medical hierarchies are convinced (probably wrongly) that their patients would never again be given admission to the beds of the Sir Lancelot Spratts of this world (Sir Lancelot Spratt was the stereotyped, overbearing London teaching hospital surgeon in Dr Richard Gordon's *Doctor in the House* book and film series).

Hopefully vocational training will make future GPs more aware of their task as patient advocates, which includes the integration of patient care. GPs need to realise that they have the advantage of seeing a moving picture of a patient's life and illness. Specialists usually see only a snapshot so it is not surprising that they are not always right and need the help of good feedback. Without this feedback it is ultimately the patient who suffers.

CONCLUSION

Mutual dissatisfaction about the content and context of written communications among GPs, specialists, and hospitals has been a frequent but low-key theme in the medical literature for many decades. One theory for the lack of improvement is that *'doctors are so inured to this failing in their colleagues that thresholds for satisfaction are low'.*[47] When a specialist receives a letter from a GP saying 'obesity please treat' and a GP receives a hospital letter eight months after the patient has been discharged, it is obvious that written communications are low on those doctors' lists of priorities and that *'doctors don't really give a damn'.*[48]

But the new millennium heralds the opportunity for better communication. Information technology is making it easier, quicker, and better organised. What is also required is the attitudinal change to regard good communication as essential for comprehensive patient care and to understand a fellow health professional's needs and wish to satisfy them. This happy day will be hastened when written communication becomes a part of all vocational training programs and its assessment an accepted part of quality assurance.[49, 50] All doctors place a high value on their medical skills and reputation as a good doctor. But we seem to need a regular reminding *'that you can always tell a good doctor by the letters he [and now she] writes'.*[51]

NOTES

Thanks are due to Dr Elizabeth Whyte, general practitioner, and Clinical Professor Timothy Welborn, endocrinologist, for their helpful suggestions.

1 Marsh, S.H. and Archer, T.J. Accuracy of general practitioner referrals to a breast clinic. *Annals of the Royal College of Surgeons of England* 1996; 78: 203–5.

2 Jones, N.P., Lloyd, I.C. and Kwartz, J. General practitioner referrals to an eye hospital: a standard referral form. *Journal of the Royal Society of Medicine* 1990; 83:770–2.

3 Newton, J., Hutchinson, A., Hayes, V., McColl, E., Mackee, L. and Holland, C. Do clinicians tell each other enough? An analysis of referral communications in two specialities. *Family Practice* 1994; 11: 15–20.

4 Jenkins, R.M. Quality of general practitioner referrals to outpatient departments: assessment by specialists and a general practitioner. *British Journal of General Practice* 1993; 43: 111–13.

5 Kuyvenhoven, M.M. and De Melker, R.A. Referrals to specialists. An exploratory investigation of referrals by 13 general practitioners to medical and surgical departments. *Scandinavian Journal of Primary Health Care* 1990; 8: 53–7.

6 Britt, H., Sayer, G.P., Miller, G.C., Charles, J., Scahill, S., Horn, F., Bhasale, A. and McGeechan, K. *General Practice Activity in Australia 1998–99.* AIHW Cat. No. GEP 2. Canberra: Australian Institute of Health and Welfare (General Practice Series 2), 25 October, 1999, 96–9.

7 Marsh, Archer, 1996.

8 McConnell, D., Butow, P.N. and Tattersall, M.H. Improving the letters we write: an exploration of doctor–doctor communication in cancer care. *British Journal of Cancer* 1999; 80: 427–37.

9 Ward, P. and Carvell, J. GPs' management of acute back pain. Referral letters are inadequate (letter). *British Medical Journal* 1996; 312: 1481.

10 Linne, Y. and Rossner, S. What is 'obesity'? An analysis of referral letters to an obesity unit. *International Journal of Obesity and Related Metabolic Disorders* 1998; 22: 1231–3.

11 Welborn, T. Inadequate referral letters. *GP—Western Australian General Practitioners Magazine.* 1999 July; 24.

12 Hodge, J.A., Jacob, A., Ford, M.J. and Munro, J.F. Medical clinic referral letters. Do they say what they mean? Do they mean what they say? *Scottish Medical Journal* 1992; 37: 179–80.

13 Jacobs, L.G. and Pringle, M.A. Referral letters and replies from orthopaedic departments: opportunities missed. *British Medical Journal* 1990; 8: 470–3.

14 Metz, G. Training needed in referring writing. *Australian Doctor* 1989 Nov 15; 52.

15 Westerman, R.F., Hull, F.M., Bezemer, P.D. and Gort, G. A study of communication between general practitioners and specialists. *British Journal of General Practice* 1990; 40: 445–9.

16 Tattersall, M.H.N., Griffin, A., Dunn, S.M., Monaghan, H., Scatchard, K. and Butow, P.N. Writing to referring doctors after a new patient consultation: what is wanted and what is contained in letters from one medical oncologist. *Australian and New Zealand Journal of Medicine* 1995; 25: 479–82.

17 Hart, J.T. *Hypertension: Community Control of High Blood Pressure.* Oxford: Radcliffe Medical Press, 1993: 208–12.

18 Schnyder, U., Feld, C., Leuthold, A. and Buddeberg, C. Reference to psychiatric consultation in the discharge letter of general hospital inpatients. *International Journal of Psychiatry in Medicine* 1997; 27: 391–402.

19 Isaac, D.R., Gijsbers, A.J., Wyman, K.T., Martyres, R.F. and Garrow, B.A. The GP–hospital interface: Attitudes of general practitioners to tertiary teaching hospitals. *Medical Journal of Australia* 1997; 166: 9–12.

20 Murtagh, J.E. A safe diagnostic strategy in general practice. *General Practice* (2nd edn). Sydney: McGraw-Hill, 1998: 125–9.

21 Cochrane, R.A., Singhal, H., Monypenny, I.J., Webster, D.J., Lyons, K. and Mansel, R.E. Evaluation of general practitioner referrals to a specialist breast clinic according to the UK national guidelines. *European Journal of Surgical Oncology* 1997; 23: 198–201.
22 AMA Code of Ethics. *Responsibilities to Patients.* Canberra. Australian Medical Association, 1996.
23 Commonwealth Department of Health and Aged Care. *Medicare Benefits Schedule Book.* Canberra: Commonwealth of Australia, 1999: 7–9.
24 Graham, P.H. Improving communications with specialists: The case of an oncology clinic. *Medical Journal of Australia* 1994; 160: 625–7.
25 Schnyder et al., 1997.
26 Rivett, D. cited in I. Torjesen, Victorian health project attacked. *Australian Doctor* 1999 Aug 27: 7.
27 Nyman, K. WA tackles the 'interface'. *Australian Family Physician* 1990; 19: 647–8.
28 Metz, 1989.
29 Hamilton, W., Round, A. and Taylor, P. Dictating clinic letters in front of the patient. Letting patients see copy of consultant's letter is being studied in trial (letter). *British Medical Journal* 1997; 314: 1416.
30 Jenkins, S., Arroll, B., Hawken, S. and Nicholson, R. Referral letters: are form letters better? *British Journal of General Practice* 1997; 47: 107–8.
31 Kamien, M. What happens when patients carry their own health summaries? *Australian Family Physician* 1988; 17: 359–63.
32 van Walraven, C., Laupacis, A., Seth, R. and Wells, G. Dictated versus database-generated discharge summaries: a randomized clinical trial. *Canadian Medical Association Journal* 1999; 160: 345–6.
33 Branger, P.J., van't Hooft, A., van der Wouden, J.C., Moorman, P.W. and van Bemmel, J.H. Shared care for diabetes: supporting communication between primary and secondary care. *International Journal of Medical Informatics* 1999; 53: 133–42.
34 Girzadas, D.V. Jr, Harwood. R.C., Dearie, J. and Garrett, S. A comparison of standardised and narrative letters of recommendation. *Academic Emergency Medicine* 1998; 5: 1101–4.
35 Ray, S., Archbold, R.A., Preston, S., Ranjadayalan, K., Suliman, A. and Timmis, A.D. Computer-generated correspondence for patients attending an open-access chest pain clinic. *Journal of the Royal College of Physicians London* 1998; 32: 420–1.
36 Wass, A.R. and Illlingworth, R.N. What information do general practitioners want about accident and emergency patients? *Journal of Accident and Emergency Medicine* 1996; 13: 406–8.
37 Eaden, J.A., Ward, B. and Mayberry, J.F. Letters should be used carefully (letter). *British Medical Journal* 1998; 316: 1831.
38 Cowper, D.M. and Lenton, S.W. Letter writing to parents following paediatric outpatient consultation: a survey of parent and GP views. *Child: Care, Health and Development* 1996; 22: 303–10.

39 Lewars, M.D. GPs can be given copies of letters sent to patients (letter). *British Medical Journal* 1998; 316: 1831.

40 Eaden et al., 1998.

41 Bailey, G., Hyde, L. and Morton, R. Sending a copy of the letter to the general practitioner also to the parents in a child development centre: does it work? *Child: Care, Health and Development* 1996; 22: 411–19.

42 Royal Australian College of General Practitioners Training Program Curriculum. (2nd edn) Melbourne; RACGP Training Program, 1999: 3–9. (Paget, N. Director of Education, Royal Australian College of Physicians, personal communication, 7 October 1999.)

43 Montalto, M. Letters to go: general practitioners' referral letters to an accident and emergency department. *Medical Journal of Australia* 1991; 155: 374–7.

44 Mathur, R., Clark, R.A., Dhillon, D.P., Winter, J.H. and Lipworth, B.J. A repeat audit of hospital discharge letters in patients admitted with acute asthma. *Scottish Medical Journal* 1997; 42: 19–21.

45 Bowie, P., Dougall, A., Brown, R., Marshall, D. Turnaround time of in-patient discharge letters: a simple system of audit. *Health Bulletin* 1996; 54: 438–40.

46 Myers, K.A., Kealy, E.J, Dojeiji, S. and Norman, G.R. Development of a rating scale to evaluate written communication skills of students. *Academic Medicine* 1999; 74 (5): 612–13.

47 Newton, J., Eccles, M. and Hutchinson, A. Communication between general practitioners and consultants: what should their letters contain? *British Medical Journal* 1992; 304: 821–4.

48 Graham, P.H. and Wilson, G. Letters from the radiation oncologist: do referring doctors give a damn? *Australasian Radiology* 1998; 42: 222–4.

49 Bowie et al., 1996.

50 Myers et al., 1999.

51 Bush, J.P. You can always tell a good doctor by the letters he writes. *Australian Family Physician* 1976; 5: 1232–5.

12

Reporting

Martin B. Van Der Weyden

'Writers, like teeth, are divided into incisors and grinders.'

Walter Bagehot

'We wish to suggest a structure for the salt deoxyribose nucleic acid (DNA).' So begins the report in the journal *Nature* on the greatest discovery in science in the twentieth century—the structure of DNA.[1] Indeed, when asked the question, 'Who received the Nobel Prize for the discovery of DNA's double helix?' most people will reply, 'Watson and Crick', the authors of this report in *Nature*. When told that the Nobel Prize for Physiology or Medicine in 1962 for the structure of DNA went to Watson, Crick, and Wilkins, the response is usually 'Wilkins who?' Causing even greater surprise to most is the revelation that the famous 1953 issue of *Nature* contains, back-to-back, three reports on the structure of DNA: that by Watson and Crick[1] followed by those of Wilkins, Stokes, and Wilson[2] and Franklin and Gosling.[3]

Why, then, did Watson and Crick become the DNA megastars and why did their report receive such overwhelming acclaim, while the two other reports and their authors were virtually relegated to historical oblivion?[4]

Answers to these questions lie at the core of effective reporting, and to examine these we will explore:

- general factors that govern effective reports; and
- how these can be used for effective communication in specific instances such as: oral presentations at scientific or clinical meetings; and written reports destined for dissemination through print or electronic publication.

As an aid in these tasks we will use the *Nature* reports as case studies for effective communication.

THE PURPOSE OF A REPORT

'I ran the paper purely for propaganda and with no other purpose.'

Lord Beaverbrook

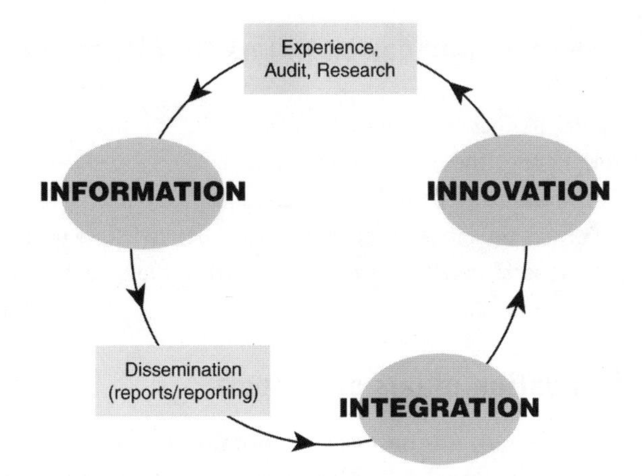

Figure 12.1 The three Is cycle

Reports and their dissemination are essential components of the information–integration–innovation (three Is) cycle (see Figure 12.1).

Information, whether acquired actively (through research or individual experience) or passively (through the specialised or popular media), influences decisions, including those made by health care professionals, researchers, providers, or policy makers.

The primary purpose of a report is to inform and influence. In order to do this, it must first be communicated and exposed to scrutiny and debate. If it is accepted as both rigorous and relevant, it will be integrated into the pool of living information, from where it has the power to influence. The secondary purpose of reports is to innovate and bring about change. This innovation in turn, is subject to further research, audit, and experience, thus completing the three Is cycle.

EFFECTIVE REPORTS

'Words are like leaves, and where they most abound
Much fruit of sense beneath is rarely found.'

Alexander Pope

If we agree that the purpose of a report is to share information in order to achieve certain outcomes, then that information has to be accessible to, and understood by, others. The report may have all the drama of Beethoven's Fifth Symphony or the grandeur of the Taj Mahal, but the beauty of these creations does not exist unless people hear the drama or see the grandeur; this applies equally to reports.

Box 12.1: The 5 W foundation pillars for effective reports

- Why the report? Defines its purpose.
- Who is it for? Defines the report's target group.
- What needs to be conveyed? Defines its content.
- What way? Defines the mode of reporting, attitude, and style of its content.
- Who owns the report? Defines the report's owner, authors, and accountability.

The five W foundation pillars of a report

Before a report is prepared, it is necessary to obtain unambiguous answers to the five questions shown in Box 12.1. Although these questions might seem self-evident, reports continue to be produced that fail to address these fundamental questions. Their answers will determine the report's content, its dissemination, and, most importantly, its attitude and style.

ATTITUDE AND STYLE OF REPORTS

> 'Have something to say and say it as clearly as you can. That is the essence of style.'
>
> Matthew Arnold

A reader or listener responds to three features of a report: its content, its presentation, and its language. The efficacy of a report is determined by its attitude—the determination of the report's creator(s) to organise and deliver information in such a way that makes minimal demands on the reader or listener—and its style—use of language that is accurate, easy to process, and appropriate in tone.[5]

Some twenty-five years ago, the *New England Journal of Medicine* featured two articles with identical titles.[6, 7] At first glance, this appeared to be an editorial glitch. Closer scrutiny, however, revealed not a blunder but a bold experiment. The editor had published back-to-back a scientific immunological article replete with technical jargon and results so complex 'as to preclude any defined concepts', and a plain English translation of the same article by a science writer. Reasons given by the journal's editor, Franz Ingelfinger, for performing such an audacious act included frustration and annoyance at the 'unfriendliness' to most readers of specialised reports.[8] This was a very public protest about the deterioration in attitude and style of reports. Despite this editor's protest, reports today continue to be characterised by an elitist attitude and pompous style, readily recognised by their tedious and verbose content, dense syntax, and technical jargon monotonously delivered in an impersonal passive voice (see Box 12.2).

Box 12.2: Examples of 'learned journalese'[9, 10]

'The mode of action of lymphocytic serum (ALS) has not yet been determined by research workers in this country or abroad.'
Change to: We don't know how ALS works.
'A high proportion of the young female population is now smoking cigarettes.
Change to: More young women now smoke cigarettes.
'It has been shown by the present author, on the basis of preliminary evidence that has not yet been independently replicated by other investigators, that an appropriate quantity of milk is absent from the refrigerator.'
Change to: I can see no milk in the fridge; can someone have a look?
'Therefore, to maximise the likelihood of a guideline being used, we need coherent dissemination and implementation strategies to capitalise on known positive factors and to deal with obstacles to implementation.'
Change to: We need to know why guidelines are used or not used, in order to increase their uptake.

In his essay 'Plain words please',[9] Bernard Dixon, the editor of *Medical Science Research*, noted that the perpetrators of this 'learned journalese' are scarcely aware of their abuse of language, and that 'many scientists never consider the contrast between their conversation over the breakfast table and the weird, stilted cadences they use to communicate with their peers.' This peculiar way of communicating reflects a culture in which reports serve the needs of their creators and their peers rather than those of the general reader—'an inherent dishonesty of writing in order to be published rather than to be read.'[10] An astute observation by George Orwell captures the essence of this culture: 'the great enemy of clear language is insincerity. When there is a gap between one's real and one's declared aims, one turns, as it were, instinctively to long words and exhausted idioms like a cuttlefish squirting ink'.[11] It needs to be continually stressed that the purpose of reports is 'to share our information and ideas in a clear, honest, and interesting way',[12] reaching out to, and involving as many people as possible. Some useful tools for effective reporting style are shown in Box 12.3.

THE WATSON AND CRICK PAPER: A CASE STUDY IN EFFECTIVE REPORTS

With this background, let us examine the Watson and Crick paper on the structure of DNA (see Box 12.4) and judge how it measures up to the determinants of effective reports.

Box 12.3: Useful tools for effective reporting style

- Keep the report short.

Readers' time and journal space are at a premium.

- Use the active voice.

It has greater impact, and is more immediate and personal.

- Keep sentences short.

Long sentences tend to discourage readers from continuing. Moreover, syntax may come adrift in sentences that are too lengthy.

- Use simple language and keep technical jargon to a minimum.

Long and overly technical words do not equate to intellectual or scientific excellence, and irritate rather than impress readers.

- Use figures and tables rather than text.

Figures and tables are worth a thousand words.

- Take care when using abbreviations.

Always spell out an abbreviation when it is first used, and try not to use too many.

Papers littered with abbreviations are difficult to read.

- Record the report aloud and then listen to it.

This identifies mistakes in syntax.

- Ask another uninvolved person to read the report.

Invite suggestions to clarify points not understood.

Box 12.4: The Watson and Crick article in *Nature*

Molecular structure of nucleic acids

A structure for deoxyribose nucleic acid

We wish to suggest a structure for the salt of deoxyribose nucleic acid (D.N.A.). This structure has novel features which are of considerable biological interest.

A structure for nucleic acid has already been proposed by Pauling and Corey.[1] They kindly made their manuscript available to us in advance of publication. Their model consists of three intertwined chains, with the phosphates near the fibre axis, and the bases on the outside. In our opinion, this structure is unsatisfactory for two reasons: (1) We believe that the material which gives the X-ray diagrams is the salt, not the free acid. Without the acidic hydrogen atoms it is not clear what forces would hold the structure together, especially as the negatively charged phosphates near the axis will repel each other. (2) Some of the van der Waals distances appear to be too small.

Another three-chain structure has also been suggested by Fraser (in the press). In his model the phosphates are on the outside and the bases on the inside, linked together by hydrogen bonds. This structure as described is rather ill-defined, and for this reason we shall not comment on it.

We wish to put forward a radically different structure for the salt of deoxyribose nucleic acid. This structure has two helical chains each coiled round the same axis (see diagram). We have made the usual chemical assumptions, namely, that each chain consists of phosphate diester groups joining β-D-deoxyribofuranose residues with 3′,5′ linkages. The two chains (but not their bases) are related by a dyad perpendicular to the fibre axis. Both chains follow right-handed helices, but owing to the dyad the sequences of the atoms in the two chains run in opposite directions. Each chain loosely resembles Furberg's[2] model No. 1; that is, the bases are on the inside of the helix and the phosphates on the outside. The configuration of the sugar and the atoms near it is close to Furberg's 'standard configuration', the sugar being roughly perpendicular to the attached base. There is a residue on each chain every 3.4 A. in the *z*-direction. We have assumed an angle of 36° between adjacent residues in the same chain so that the structure repeats after 10 residues on each chain, that is, after 34 A. The distance of a phosphorus atom from the fibre axis is 10 A. As the phosphates are on the outside, cations have easy access to them.

The structure is an open one, and its water content is rather high. At lower water contents we would expect the bases to tilt so that the structure could become more compact.

The novel feature of the structure is the manner in which the two chains are held together by the purine and pyrimidine bases. The planes of the bases are perpendicular to the fibre axis. They are joined together in pairs, a single base from one chain being hydrogen-bonded to a single base from the other chain, so that the two lie side by side with identical z-coordinates. One of the pair must be a purine and the other a pyrimidine for bonding to occur. The hydrogen bonds are made as follows: purine position 1 to pyrimidine position 1; purine position 6 to pyrimidine position 6.

If it is assumed that the bases only occur in the structure in the most plausible tautomeric forms (that is, with the keto rather than the enol configurations) it is found that only specific pairs of bases can bond together. These pairs are: adenine (purine) with thymine (pyrimidine), and guanine (purine) with cytosine (pyrimidine).

In other words, if an adenine forms one member of a pair, on either chain, then on these assumptions the other member must be thymine; similarly for guanine and cytosine. The sequence of bases on a single chain does not appear to be restricted in any way. However, if only specific pairs of bases can be formed, it follows that if the sequence of bases on one chain is given, then the sequence on the other chain is automatically determined.

It has been found experimentally[3, 4] that the ratio of the amounts of adenine to thymine, and the ratio of the amounts of guanine to cytosine, are always very close to unity for deoxyribose nucleic acid.

It is probably impossible to build this structure with a ribose sugar in place of the deoxyribose, as the extra oxygen atom would make too close a van der Waals contact.

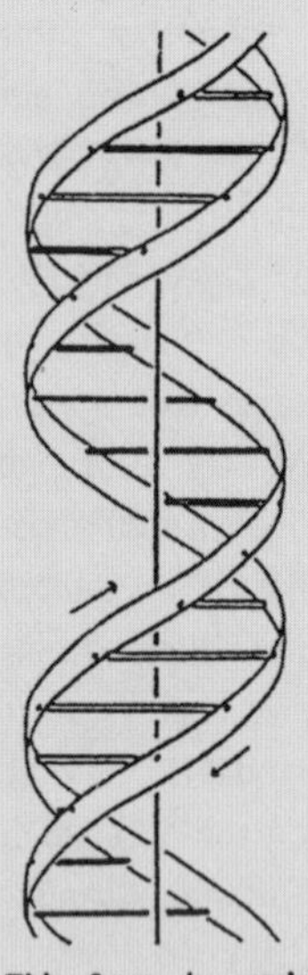

This figure is purely diagrammatic. The two ribbons symbolize the two phosphate—sugar chains, and the horizontal rods the pairs of bases holding the chains together. The vertical line marks the fibre axis

The previously published X-ray data[5, 6] on deoxyribose nucleic acid are insufficient for a rigorous test of our structure. So far as we can tell, it is roughly compatible with the experimental data, but it must be regarded as unproved until it has been checked against more exact results. Some of these are given in the following communications. We were not aware of the details of the results presented there when we devised our structure, which rests mainly although not entirely on published experimental data and stereochemical arguments.

It has not escaped our notice that the specific pairing we have postulated immediately suggests a possible copying mechanism for the genetic material.

Full details of the structure, including the conditions assumed in building it, together with a set of coordinates for the atoms, will be published elsewhere.

We are much indebted to Dr Jerry Donohue for constant advice and criticism, especially on interatomic distances. We have been stimulated by a knowledge of the general nature of the unpublished experimental results and ideas of Dr M H F Wilkins, Dr R E Franklin and their co-workers at King's College, London. One of us (JDW) has been aided by a fellowship from the National Foundation for Infantile Paralysis.

J. D. WATSON

F. H. C. CRICK

Medical Research Council Unit for the Study of the Molecular Structure of Biological Systems, Cavendish Laboratory, Cambridge, April 2.

1 Pauling L., and Corey, R. B., *Nature*, 171, 346 (1953); *Proc. U.S. Nat. Acad. Sci.*, 39, 84 (1953).

2 Furberg, S., *Acta Chem. Scand.*, 6, 634 (1952).

3 Chargaff, E., for references see Zamenhof, S., Brawerman, G., and Chargaff, E., *Biochim. et Biophys. Acta*, 9, 402 (1952).
4 Wyatt, G. R., *J. Gen. Physiol.*, 36, 201 (1952).
5 Astbury, W.T., *Symp. Soc. Exp. Biol. 1, Nucleic Acid*, 66 (Camb. Univ. Press, 1947).
6 Wilkins, M. H. F., and Randall, J.T., *Biochim. et Biophys. Acta*, 10, 192 (1953).

Adherence to the foundation pillars of reports

Why the report?

Its purpose is stated in its simple opening sentence: 'We wish to suggest a structure for the salt deoxyribose nucleic acid'—no ambiguity here!

Who is it for?

Although not explicitly stated in the report, choosing to submit their article to the journal *Nature* (which was science's most prestigious forum at the time) suggests that Watson and Crick aimed to reach as many scientists as possible. Further, the report's tenor suggests that they were targeting people well beyond the scientific world.

What needs to be conveyed?

This is clearly identified by the statement: 'We wish to put forward a radically different structure for the salt deoxyribose nucleic acid'. Watson and Crick did this by clearly describing their evidence for their proposed structure. The effectiveness of their report also shows that it is best to address one or two themes rather than overwhelming the reader with distracting information that is not directly relevant.

What way is it conveyed?

Watson and Crick's report is brief, and uses the active voice and simple language with minimal technical jargon. The central message of the report is illustrated by a simple diagram showing the double helix of DNA. The report concludes with the prescient statement: 'It has not escaped our notice that the specific pairing we have postulated suggests a possible copying mechanism for the genetic material', which signals to the world the significance of their discovery.

Who owns the report?

The intellectual property is clearly identified as that of Watson and Crick, although they acknowledge the unpublished experimental results and ideas [*sic*] of the senior authors of the reports that followed their paper.

Attitude and style of the report

It is easy to understand why the Watson and Crick paper is a classic among scientific reports. It is brief—only 950 words, occupying only one page of the journal. Its active voice uses clear English prose and the report is almost devoid of any technical jargon—it is inclusive. The efficacy of the paper's style becomes even more obvious when compared with the reports of Wilkins, Stokes, and Wilson,[13] and Franklin and Gosling.[14] These reports are both twice as long as the Watson and Crick report, they are delivered in the dull passive voice and their tenor is exclusive, their language abounding with 'arcane jargon; it was as if they took joy in befuddling the reader with esoteric physical-chemical data'.[15] In stark contrast to the simple ink drawing illustrating the Watson and Crick paper, both reports contain highly specialised and poorly defined X-ray diffraction pictures (either badly reproduced or so complex as to be beyond most readers). These papers, although undoubtedly of the highest scientific quality, do not have the attributes of effective reports: brevity, clarity, conciseness, and inclusiveness.

Pre-eminence of the Watson and Crick report

Why then are Watson and Crick synonymous with the structure of DNA while Wilkins, Stokes, and Wilson, and Franklin and Gosling are practically unknowns? The holy grail of science is to be first in discovery. Although the three reports on the structure of DNA appeared in the same issue of *Nature*, the fact that Watson and Crick's paper preceded the others gives it the perceived status of being first. Watson's subsequent personal account of the excitement of the race leading up to publication[16] undoubtedly played a publicity role, but overriding all of this is the effect of the marked difference in the attitude and style of the three reports.

EFFECTIVE REPORTING

> 'It is said that writing becomes more easy if you have something to say.'
>
> Shalem Asch

Now that we have explored what constitutes an effective report, we will examine factors that govern effective communication—the dissemination link of the three I's cycle (Figure 12.1)—either through oral communication (usually to peers) or written communication (through stand-alone publications, favoured by bureaucratic organisations and educational bodies, or through established publication forums like journals).

Barriers to effective reporting

> 'We spend our midday sweat, our midnight oil;
> We tire the night in thought, the day in toil.'
>
> Francis Quarles

There are many barriers to effective reporting some of which are beyond the control of a report's creator(s). These include:

- limited interest, even among peers. This disturbing phenomenon reflects the impact of microspecialisation within individual health care specialties (e.g. hepatology in gastroenterology, indigenous health in public health, intensive care specialists or community specialists in nursing)
- limited personal opportunities to read or listen to reports because of increasing pressures and call on professionals' time, and
- overwhelming information as a result of the inexorable growth of information and information technologies (one commentator recently likened the quest of professionals to keep up with information as 'trying to drink water from a fire hose').[17]

At any scientific or professional meeting, individual presentations may compete with more than a hundred other presentations spread across concurrent sessions. If published, the report will compete for attention among the more than 75 000 articles published in biomedical journals each week,[18] and the other reports that pile up in the in-trays of health professionals, including practice guidelines, medical tabloids, pharmaceutical promotions, and directives from health authorities.[19]

How, then, do we compete in the information morass?

The five W structural pillars of reporting

> 'Begin with an arresting sentence; close with a strong summary; in between speak simply and always to the point: and above all be brief.'
>
> William J. Mayo

In constructing an effective report, it is helpful to consider five 'W' structural pillars for effective reporting, shown in Box 12.5. These are based on Bradford-Hill's advice in writing a scientific papers,[20] but equally applicable to oral communication. Further, the first four questions in this Box are Bradford Hill's four fundamentals of scientific writing, to which I have added, 'What will we do with it?'

Answers to these questions will delineate the structure and content of a report, its relevance, and will also promote a realistic approach to selecting the

Box 12.5: The five W structural pillars of reporting

- What did we do?
  Defines the outcomes of a report and the methods used to determine the outcomes.
- Why did we do what we did?
  Defines the introduction of the report.
- What did we find?
  Defines the results of the outcome measures of the report.
- What does it mean?
  Defines the context of the report in relation to previous findings and what actions are appropriate outcomes.
- What will we do with it?
  Defines the reporting vehicle: oral or written.

vehicle for reporting. The use of the five pillars of reports and of reporting is illustrated in Figure 12.2.

SELECTING A FORUM FOR REPORTING

Forums for oral reporting are usually predetermined. For example, the report may be an audit or a paper to be presented to peers or to members of a professional body or scientific society. More difficult is choosing a peer-reviewed biomedical or other journal, of which there are more than 20 000![21] The critical question is 'what journal do I wish to report my report?' To answer this will require a brief aside to examine the nature of peer-review journals.

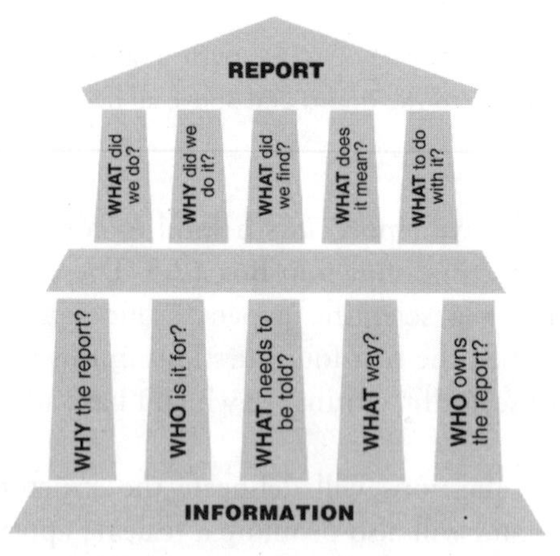

Figure 12.2 The pillars of reports and reporting

Almost forty years ago, Sir Theodore Fox, editor of the *Lancet*, in his Heath–Clark lectures on the function and future of (peer-review) medical journals, divided journals in two major categories—recorder (specialist) and newspaper (general) journals.[22] The former publish new observations, experiments, and techniques and exist principally to record advances in medical knowledge. The role of general medical journals is to inform, interpret, criticise, and stimulate, and they exist to advance the practice of medicine. Today, despite the roll-out of electronic publications, this concept is still relevant.

At one extreme of the journal spectrum are specialist journals that cater for a specific group bound by a special purpose; such journals are usually journals of record tinged with conservatism and elitism. At the other extreme is the general journal, which besides being a journal of record is a journal of opinion walking a tightrope balancing conservatism with a subversive streak and its responsibilities to professional groups and to society. Most journals are hybrids of these two extremes and it is the editor of a journal who has to manage and blend these competing forces in satisfying its authors and readers.

Reporting priorities of authors and journals

> 'Unfortunately too many authors write as though they will never get another chance—and unfortunately they are correct.'
>
> M. Therese Southgate

Authors and journals have different reasons for publishing (see Box 12.6), which sometimes lead to conflict and misunderstanding. It is important to remember that each journal has its own character and style. A common reason

Box 12.6: Reasons for reporting

Authors

Why do I want to report this?

- important information to communicate
- add to knowledge
- peer approval
- career advancement
- secure or protect funding
- pressure from above, i.e. the boss

Publishers

Why should we publish this?

- who will read this?
- is it important for the knowledge base and/or delivery of health care in the community?
- how original and rigorous is the report?
- is it easy to read and comprehend?

for editors deciding not to publish a report is not the report *per se*, but the incongruity between the attitude and style of the report and that of the journal. It is therefore extremely important to read a journal and be familiar with its individual character and style before submitting an article.

PRACTICAL POINTERS FOR ORAL AND WRITTEN REPORTS

> 'If I am to speak for ten minutes, I need a week for preparation: if fifteen minutes, three days; if half an hour two days; if an hour, I am ready now.'
>
> Woodrow Wilson

Box 12.7: Useful pointers for reporting

Verbal reporting

- Be familiar with the venue (e.g. the room, podium, and audience seating) and reporting facilities (e.g. audiovisual equipment).
- Basic presentation rules: observe the time limit; leave time for questions; have simple audiovisual aids (e.g. overheads, slides, Powerpoint, which should be readable and easy to understand); have backups in case of facility failure; have at least two jokes in reserve; keep the visual aids simple, brief, and to the point.
- Audience involvement—attitude and style: memorise the presentation and avoid merely reading from personal notes; maintain eye contact with the audience; never be in a situation that requires the prefaces: 'I am sorry you cannot read this, but ...'; 'I know this is a busy diagram/overhead/slide, but ...'; 'This diagram may be complex, but ...'; and finally do not read the visual aids—the audience can do this just as well!

Written reporting

- Conform to the five structural 'pillars' of reporting.
- Select the appropriate vehicle for publishing (e.g. specialist or general journal).
- Respect the publication's requirements: read the journal or previous reports from the publisher; and read the guidelines to contributors and comply with them.
- Adhere to requirements for individual articles, such as papers on research, systematic reviews, case reports, etc.
- Remember to be brief, clear, and concise, and ensure that the recommendations reflect the content of the paper.

The specifics of publishing and writing for publication are detailed elsewhere (chapters 16 and 17), but some generic guides for both oral and written reporting are shown in Box 12.7. There is a plethora of format guidelines for both forms of reporting, but most do not cover the essential ingredient of ensuring an appropriate attitude and style.

It is hoped that this concise explanation of these attributes of effective reporting will increase your ability to communicate with people through reports and reporting. Irrespective of whether your report is an oral or written communication, an excellent piece of advice to keep in mind is that

> Writing when properly managed ... is but a different name for conversation.
>
> (Laurence Sterne).

NOTES

1 Watson, J.O. and Crick, O.H. A structure for deoxyribose nucleic acid. *Nature* 1953; 171: 737–8.

2 Wilkins, M.H.F., Stokes, A.R. and Wilson, H.R. Molecular structure of deoxypentose nucleic acids. *Nature* 1953; 171: 738–40.

3 Franklin, R.Y.E. and Gosling, R.U.G. Molecular configuration in sodium thymonucleate. *Nature* 1953; 171: 740–2.

4 Friedman, M. and Freidlander, G.O. *Medicine's 10 Greatest Discoveries*. New Haven, Conn.: Yale University Press, 1998: 192–227.

5 Kirkman, J. Writing well. Presentation at BMJ/EASE Workshop for editors of journals. Tunbridge Wells, United Kingdom: 9–10 November 1995. (An abridged version was published in *European Science Editing* 1996; 57: 6–7, with commentary by M. Grace: 7–8).

6 Gutterman, J.U., Rosen, R.D., Butler, W.T., McCredie, K.B., Body G.P., Sr. Freireich and Hersh, E.M. Immunoglobulin on tumor cells and tumor-induced lymphocyte blastogenesis in human acute leukemia. [Revision by B.J. Culliton.] *New England Journal of Medicine* 1973; 288: 169–73.

7 Gutterman, J.U., Rosen, R.D. Butler, W.T., McCredie, K.B., Body G.P., Sr. Freireich and Hersh, E.M. Immunoglobulin on tumor cells and tumor-induced lymphocyte blastogenesis in human acute leukemia. [Revision by B.J. Culliton.] *New England Journal of Medicine* 1973; 288: 173–5.

8 Ingelfinger, F.J. Twin bill on tumor immunity [editorial]. *New England Journal of Medicine* 1973; 288: 211.

9 Dixon, B. Plain words please. *New Scientist* 1993; 137: 39–40.

10 O'Donnell, M. Evidence-based illiteracy: time to rescue the literature. *Lancet* 2000; 355: 489–91.

11 Orwell, G. *Politics and the English: Inside the Whale and Other Essays.* London: Penguin, 1957: 154.

12 O'Donnell, 2000.
13 Wilkins et al., 1953.
14 Franklins, Gosling, 1953.
15 Friedman, Friedlander, 1998.
16 Watson, J.O. *The Double Helix: A Personal Account of the Discovery of the Structure of DNA.* London: Penguin, 1968.
17 Wallet, R.R. Tomorrow's challenges and opportunities. *Mayo Clinic Proceedings* 2000; 75: 981–2.
18 Bernier, C.L. and Yerkey, A.N. *Cogent Communication.* Westport, Conn.: Greenwich Press, 1979: 39.
19 Hobble, A., Sanka, D., Poinciana, D. and Pools, F. Guidelines in general practice. *British Medical Journal* 1998; 317: 862–3.
20 Anonymous. The reason for writing. *British Medical Journal* 1965; 2: 870–2.
21 O'Donnell, 2000.
22 Fox, T.F. *Crisis in Communication: The Functions and Future of Medical Journals.* London: Athlone Press, 1965.

13

Teams that work

Marianne Hammerton, Paul Sadler, and Alan Cartwright

The focus of this chapter is communication within a team. A successful team is often multidisciplinary, and is able to work on complex issues effectively and efficiently. This chapter draws on a case study of the development of cross-organisational teams in the community health context, analysing it from a theoretical and practical point of view. Group work theory is used to analyse the operations of teams and to provide an outline of how to make them work. Some exercises that can be used at various stages of team development are included because they work and, moreover, they can be fun! Finally, we examine why making teams work matters, with reference to the outcomes of the case study and its implications for health care professionals.

Try this exercise first of all.

Box 13.1: 'Team Assessment' Quiz

Take two sheets of blank paper.

1. Recall a team you have been part of that did not seem to work well, or was not an enjoyable group to be part of. On one sheet make a list of all the reasons why, in hindsight, you think that team or group *did not work so well*. What is your assessment?
2. Recall a team you have been part of that worked well and that you enjoyed being part of. On the other sheet, make a list of all the reasons why, in hindsight, you think the team or group *worked well*. What is your assessment?

N.B. If you have been in neither ask a colleague to volunteer their experience and make some notes about their answers to 1 and 2 above.

Keep this information handy as at the end of this chapter you will reassess it in light of what you have read and we will use it to consolidate your learning.

TEAMS IN HEALTH CARE

Those of us who work in health care have a commitment to improving client and/or patient care. It is a given that to achieve improved health outcomes for individuals, professionals need to work collectively. This chapter is provided for you to build on your understanding of what makes successful teams work.

Successful results involving the interaction of people are most likely to come from those groups that have a common intention and a strong, workable sense of team interplay. Many teams form quite naturally and are spectacular in their performance and results. Others too form, but somehow miss the mark, often being consumed by factors such as unclear direction, squabbling over roles and responsibilities, and presumed 'scarce' resources. This applies to teams in many organisational and industry contexts, including health.

It is rare for health care professionals to operate in complete isolation from other professionals, let alone the patients with whom they work. Even where practitioners have a single-person practice, such as a GP in a remote rural area, or a chiropractor operating a sole practice, they have to work collaboratively with other professionals, such as specialists to whom they refer. In most health care contexts, working with a multidisciplinary team is essential. For example, a hospital ward involves medical practitioners, nurses, allied health professionals, and other ward staff while specialist multidisciplinary teams are seen as an asset in community contexts, such as mental health and aged care. Many writers support the involvement of the patient and their family or other informal carers as part of the team making decisions about patient care.

As the number of health and community care providers has increased, there has been a growing interest in methods to coordinate service provision to vulnerable populations.[1] Unlike residential or acute care services, where nearly all of a person's needs are provided by the one organisation, in many community care settings multiple providers are involved, particularly for people with complex needs. The multiplicity of providers can cause problems for people needing services, who experience difficulties accessing services and duplication in assessment procedures.[2, 3] Forming a team that works across these organisational boundaries is a particular challenge.

CASE STUDY—NEW SOUTH WALES COMMUNITY CARE DEMONSTRATION PROJECTS

The process of developing demonstration projects on integrated community care services in the most highly populated state in Australia, New South Wales, commenced in 1992. The aim of these projects was to systematically trial and evaluate models of community care that replace fragmented and overspecialised services with more coherent local service delivery arrangements. The projects examined how effective different local models are in bringing about the desired changes. The main objectives of the community care demonstration projects were to assess the ability of alternative funding and service arrangements to:

- enhance consumer outcomes
- improve service delivery, including assessment, case management, coordination, support for carers, targeting, and responsiveness to individual clients, and
- encourage development of the most cost-effective services.[4, 5]

Three models were developed following a consultation process undertaken by a state government agency, the Office on Ageing.[6] The models sought to address issues and to build on the strengths of the current system. Expressions of interest were sought in 1994 from health or community care agencies prepared to work collaboratively to trial one of the models outlined in Table 13.1 (p. 166) in their area.

In November 1994, ten areas were selected to undertake further work on their models and to begin being evaluated. No area proceeded with the area budget holder model. Subsequently a variant of this model has been trialled by the Commonwealth Department of Health and Aged Care via the Coordinated Care Trials. By 1995, eight areas across New South Wales (four in metropolitan Sydney and four in regional New South Wales) had decided to continue into the implementation phase of their projects. Implementation continued until June 1998.

Four areas were evaluated in depth by the Social Policy Research Centre, University of New South Wales (Manly–Warringah–Pittwater, Sutherland, Orange–Cabonne, and Tamworth) and a further four participated in data collection (Baulkham Hills, Ryde–Hunters Hill, Ballina–Byron, and Wagga Wagga). The evaluation results show that in each project, *working together as a team* across traditional health and community care boundaries was a key ingredient to the success or otherwise of the new model. Each of the projects formed a local steering committee involving a range of health and community care service providers and often consumer representatives. These largely operated on a consensus decision-making model, making effective teamwork vital. Further details of the evaluation can be found in Fine et al.[7] and *Community Solutions.*[8]

THEORETICAL APPROACHES TO COORDINATION AND GROUP PROCESSES

We will now consider some of the theories that explain the structural and interpersonal aspects of making teams work.

Table 13.1: Models proposed for Demonstration Projects

Model	*Description*
Mandated Cooperation	Under this model, the best elements of cooperation that already exist in the community care system are given a more formal status. Local service providers and agencies draw up written agreements about how they can best cater for the needs of consumers. Ideally, these written agreements introduce common assessment protocols and lead to reduction of service duplication and to consistent pricing policies. They are also designed to allow service providers more flexibility in meeting consumer needs. Providers may, for example offer new types of services or provide services outside normal working hours. Funding bodies set clear guidelines for their agreements with service providers and both parties negotiate a way of evaluating whether they have met their obligations.
Integrated Community Care Agency	The Integrated Community Care Agency is a 'one-stop shop' for consumers. It offers a single phone number and premises that become the first point of entry for consumers to the community care system in their local area. The lead agency negotiates agreements with service providers in the local area—whether they are housed within the agency premises or outside—about assessment of consumer needs and referral procedures. Housing community care services together paves the way for sharing overheads such as administrative time, office equipment, reception costs, and so forth. Savings made in these areas can then be channelled back into the provision of services. The lead agency model does not affect funding arrangements—funding continues to come from the relevant government departments.
Area-based Budget Holder	The budget holder is a regional authority set up to oversee the mix of publicly funded community services in a local area. It would hold the funds that the relevant state and Commonwealth departments now allocate to community service providers for aged and disability programs. The focus might initially be on funds for managed care for high or complex needs clients. The budget holder negotiates contracts with local service providers and these contracts specify the mix and volume of services to be delivered and the price and quality of services. Ideally, the budget holder encourages the delivery of quality services in a way that best meets the needs of consumers and carers.

Coordination

The concept of coordination for aged and community care services is difficult to define. Fine et al. identify a continuum of coordination in human services, moving from autonomy through cooperation and coordination to integration.[9] This continuum is represented in Figure 13.1.

⇐ **Integration**

Autonomy ⇒

Autonomy	Cooperation	Coordination	Integration
Parties/agencies act without reference to each other, although the actions of one may affect the other(s).	Parties show a willingness to work together for some common goals. Communication is emphasised. Requires development of a 'degree of goodwill and mutual understanding'.	Planned harmonisation of activities between the separate parties. Duplication of activities and resources is minimised. Requires agreed plans and protocols or appointment of a third party coordinator or (case) manager.	Links between the separate parties begin to draw them into a single system. Boundaries between parties begin to dissolve, as they become effectively work units or sub-groups within a single, larger organisation.

Source: Fine et al. 1998

Figure 13.1 The concept of coordination: a basic schema

Most health and community service organisations are established as separate entities. In health care, there has been a strong trend to specialisation linked to particular professional expertise. Similarly, many community services have been established over the past twenty years around particular areas of expertise, for example home modifications or respite care. However, consumers of health and community care services can find the multiplicity of separate providers confusing and sometimes resent the multiple assessments that they have to undergo.

This raises the importance of coordination between providers for the benefit of their consumers. In many cases, informal arrangements have existed for many years and qualify as cooperation in the schema in Figure 13.1. More recently, the importance of establishing more formal arrangements has been stressed. The idea is that these protocols or other formal arrangements are less reliant on individual personalities than informal cooperation and should therefore ensure ongoing commitment to practices that benefit people who use services. Beyond this, agencies may move to more formal integration, possibly involving establishment of cross-agency teams or amalgamation of agency management.

Group processes

A key to understanding how to work with teams of health and community service professionals is to understand how groups of people work. Tuckman identified five main stages that groups move through in their evolution and development over time: forming, norming, performing, storming, and adjourning as shown in Table 13.2.[10, 11]

Table 13.2: Stages of Group Development

Stage of group development	*Description*
Forming	In the forming stage, group members learn about each other and the task at hand. They feel 'safe' to be in the team being built and generate a sense of unity.
Norming	During the norming stage, group members establish implicit or explicit rules about how they will achieve their goal and indeed agree on the goal. They address the types of communication that will or will not help with the task.
Performing	In the performing stage, group members implement the decisions made.
Storming	As group members become more comfortable with each other, they will engage each other in arguments and vie for status in the group. These activities mark the storming phase. If healthy, they will focus on seeking clarity of tasks to be performed and not be driven by personality or relationships.
Adjourning	As the group project ends, the group disbands in the adjournment phase. Success is usually acknowledged and a degree of celebration ideally occurs.

Adapted from: Tuckman[12] and Tuckman & Jensen[13]

Many people make the mistake of not allowing time for the team to do its *forming* and *norming*. Often, the practical task-focused nature of many health and community settings is reflected in the practitioners who 'just want to get on with' the task at hand—that is, move straight to performing. An example of this is people drawing up agendas for first meetings of groups that list all the tasks that need to be done. This is clearly a *performing* stage—members of the group are likely to resist and ask questions like 'when did we agree to this?' Such responses are not a useful starting point for a team and are more likely to generate the unhealthy aspect of storming, that is, conflict rather than harmony.

The Tuckman model, by identifying the various stages of group development, assists those seeking to work with teams to understand what actions you can take at strategic moments to achieve successful outcomes. This model does not assume groups always move sequentially through the five stages. For example, *performing* and *storming* can often be interchanged. The model, by identifying five clear stages that groups or teams move through in their life cycle, allows us:

- the opportunity to identify and therefore understand the particular stage of a group's development or life cycle
- to identify processes, interventions, and conversations that will either cement or clarify a particular stage and pave the way for the group to progress comfortably to the next stage, and
- to increase enormously the likely sense of team and individual commitment and effort that 'members' contribute to the team.

This of course increases the team's success or outputs.

THE STAGES IN PRACTICE

Let's break down the stages and, using some exercises, build our insights into the process of making teams work.

Forming

The forming stage focuses on building the team and becoming familiar with the history and experience of the others on the team. This lays the platform for trust required to make the next stage work.

Desired outcomes are for team members to:

- feel welcome and included
- know who other team members are and their respective histories, and
- feel 'safe' to participate in the group.

Process exercises for forming

'About me': either seated or standing. Ask each person in the group to give their name, an overview of their background, where they live and what they are expecting to get from being on the team.

Name tags: given that not everyone will remember everyone's name, a fun exercise is to give the group blank name tags and coloured pens and ask them to go and find someone in the room they do not know. They should introduce themselves to that person and then make a name tag for them to wear during the session with just their first name. Tell them to be as creative as possible using multiple colours.

'Three things about me': ask each member of the group in turn to state three things about them that the rest of the group would not know. Two of the things must be the truth and one must be a lie. The group then has to guess which is the lie and why. This is always a lot of fun.

Norming

The norming stage involves clarifying the shared goals, their parameters, and their consequences and implications. A strong sense of team focus or purpose is defined here; what the team is aiming to achieve. This is where protocols for the team's operations are established, including clarification of roles and responsibilities of team members. In this stage the communication processes are established that will keep the team on track and communicating well.

Desired outcomes are to have:

- identified a purpose or goal
- defined our values and/or code of behaviour
- agreed major objectives or milestones
- agreed on roles and responsibilities
- agreed communication mechanisms and milestones including frequency of team meeting
- agreed evaluation or monitoring mechanisms, and
- formulated a possible project plan in draft.

Process exercises for norming

Our purpose: ask the group to define and agree on what it thinks its purpose is. Why do we exist, what is it we are here to do? Do not underestimate the significance of this process. It will set the overall direction for the group. Consider, for instance, what differing courses of action might follow depending on how the question 'are we here to care for illness or wellness?' is answered. This process must involve the entire team and requires people to agree on and understand the meaning of and significance of the words.

1 Ask each member to take a piece of paper and write on it their understanding of the team's purpose—what is it we are here to do? Why do we exist? (This may take people five to ten minutes. Ask them to work by themselves). Some people may want a simple statement, others may like to draw a picture, others may want to write some key words. (If the terms of reference have been set get the group to explore their interpretation of what they think their purpose is.)
2 Then ask people in groups of, say, five to six to report back to that group and agree on a common purpose based on the ideas they have already generated (this could take fifteen to twenty minutes).
3 If there are several groups then of course restate each of the groups' purpose statements to the large group and agree. It is important here to give this process time to make sure people have conversations to understand the meanings of words.
4 Tip: Whiteboard and butcher's paper work well here!

A useful metaphor to use with the groups while they are developing the 'concept' of their purpose is to keep stating: 'In the first case we just want to get into the right paddock, not the particular blade of grass at this point.' This stops group members being pedantic about particular words at this stage.

Our values or guiding principles: teams need to overtly agree their values or guiding principles—the things they agree to stand and work by. (Values can be defined as the things people will fight to prevent being violated or are passionate about.) Ask each individual to list the three most important values that they think the team needs to have and then pool them to agree on a final list. Ideally you need to work the data to come up with a list of a maximum of six to seven key values.

Our code of behaviour: This is a much more practical translation of the team values in action. The code of behaviour will usually include really simple things, for example, that meetings start and finish on time or 'do not shoot the messenger'. The best way to generate the code is to ask the group this question using the above examples—'If we were to develop and agree how we should work together successfully and be respectful of each other, what are some of the things we would need to do?'

Performing

The performing stage is about getting the job done; working through the agreed actions of the team both as individuals and collectively.

Desired outcomes are:

- completion of the tasks or the work
- communication and updating about work progress, and
- keeping the team members included and acknowledged for their ongoing contribution.

Process check for performing

There are no set processes to observe here except to ensure that all successfully performing teams have the following in place:

- *a reconnection process*: this is where the team meetings are allowed to start informally. This might be over a cup of tea or people simply stating how it has been going so far before any formal agenda is commenced.
- *agendas for meetings*
- *a good chairperson*
- *effective listening in place*
- *people asking more questions and making fewer statements*: this fosters exploration and consideration
- *recognition processes,* in which the group is asked at the end of the meeting to acknowledge collectively what they are proud of so far.

Storming

The storming stage will vary according to how well the *forming* and *norming* stages were done. If they were done poorly or overlooked completely the 'conflict' in the storming stage has the risk of making the team dysfunctional. The conflict in this stage that is healthy is usually about role clarification and responsibilities and can strengthen relationships. Trust and confidence built in the *forming* and *norming* stages will allow healthy conflict to occur in a respectful and trusting way. Disputes in this stage will usually be about unaddressed or agreed norming issues that are only now surfacing. The desired outcome is simply to resolve storming or conflict with clarity and agreement. It may be that the agreement reached is to disagree.

Process exercises for storming

It is assumed that if the forming and norming is done well, then the likelihood of storming is reduced. Early warning signs to look for conflict brewing might be people not speaking up at meetings, people sniping either to or about each other, or out and out conflict. The processes below are suggested to both head off and defuse storming.

It does not matter that you may either be the leader or a participant in the group. Either way these processes will work and in our experience if you present your reading of the situation, others in the group will either agree and thereby commence the process for you—or hopefully report that all is well and things are on track and the group can move on. The following questions may be asked: 'Where are we off track and on track (as a team or on this project)?' By posing this question to the group an opportunity is provided for people to externalise their thoughts, feelings, and observations. The off-track list is then used to plan what must now be solved.

'How are we feeling?' Simply ask the group one at a time to state how they are feeling. This can be about how the team is working or how they feel about being on the team. It can be about anything they feel. Any simmering tensions will surface and provide you with the platform to resolve them, particularly if the team's values and code of behaviour reflect this.

Adjourning

The adjourning stage involves debriefing on how the task went and, most importantly, celebrating the achievements of the team and acknowledging the contribution of all members.

Desired outcomes include:

- bringing the team to a close
- reviewing/evaluating success and opportunities for next time
- celebrating the team effort, and
- farewelling each other.

Process exercises for adjourning

Outcomes check: ask the group, 'Did we achieve the purpose we set out to achieve?', drawing on sources of information that include the views of clients. This can be a process that is relatively informal right through to more formal, external independent evaluation. Powerful teams have the capacity to self-evaluate. Also ask: 'What would we do differently next time?' This allows the group to identify improvement opportunities for another time.

Recognition: ask the team on one of its agendas to plan how it thinks it should recognise its achievements. Ideally generate ideas that recognise the team, not individuals.

Celebrate: the team should determine this or appoint a group to decide this and organise the event or celebration. Even team members who have dropped out for whatever reason should be included if possible. It is important to avoid using time and business as reasons not to do this well. Ideally think of something the group does not normally do, something out of the routine, for example a lunchtime picnic, a night out at an Italian café.

WHY DOES MAKING TEAMS WORK MATTER?

Let us examine what happened in the case study. In short the evaluation of the community care demonstration projects indicates the effectiveness of a teamwork approach to the provision of health and community care services.

Perhaps the most critical component of success was a shared vision from participants in each demonstration project. This was a joint desire to improve the health and community care services available to people in their area. Trust was built between participants largely because of joint agreement to work together for the benefit of consumers.

Another key factor was the role of a key leader or small group of leaders in promoting the demonstration project locally. In all cases, one or more people took on the primary role in organising the committee meetings, gaining cooperation from other service providers, and promoting the project to the wider community.

A third common factor underlying success was an agreement to work on modest, achievable work plans. The projects that were most successful were those that set their goals modestly.

There were, for many projects, significant histories of conflict among local service providers, particularly across the health/community care divide. These conflicts meant that the storming phase of team work often involved attempts to resolve long-standing disagreements and professional jealousies. The demonstration projects did not eliminate these problems, but the trust and understanding developed by the shared vision of improving outcomes for consumers meant that considerable progress was made in some areas.

Fine et al. identify the following successful outcomes from the demonstration projects:

- significant improvements in the levels of communication and cooperation between services
- improved access for consumers to services
- revised assessment and referral procedures

- enhanced systems of referral documentation
- introduction of common policies and procedures for the coordination of care for individual clients, largely through 'At Risk' committees in rural and regional areas and case-management-type care coordination approaches in the metropolitan areas
- opportunities for greater consumer participation, and
- trialling and introduction of computerised information systems.[14]

Some of these initiatives are now being implemented throughout the community care system in New South Wales. The NSW Community Care Assessment Framework has adopted a number of the strategies developed by various demonstration projects.[15] For example, the 'Key Worker' model, whereby a service provider agrees to be appointed by the service network as a key worker for identified consumers and also agrees to perform certain tasks as a part of that role, has been adopted from the Manly–Warringah–Pittwater and Tamworth demonstration projects.

Another example was the Orange–Cabonne demonstration project, which developed a detailed assessment record that could be completed by any of the services in the local network. Three levels of assessment were identified. The first level involves completion of the Client Information and Referral Record (CIARR), which occurs for all community care consumers. The second level consists of the detailed assessment record developed by the project. This detailed record is completed by the community care health service that happens to be the client's first point of contact with the community care system. If a more complex assessment is required, then consumers are referred to specialist assessors in the health or disability systems.

A particular initiative of national significance was the development of a computer software version of the CIARR by the Manly–Warringah–Pittwater demonstration project. This software enabled the exchange of referral data between service providers via the Internet. The Client Referral System software has undergone further development since the conclusion of the demonstration project and is now in use throughout New South Wales and in some other states of Australia.

As for the impact on clients, what did the evaluation show? One concern could be that the time involved in working collaboratively in the manner undertaken by the demonstration projects might have reduced the time available for direct service delivery in each area. In fact, the demonstration project initiatives occurred at the same time as providers involved in the demonstration projects reported a 31 per cent increase in the number of hours of direct service delivery. This compared to a static level of increase in hours of service across the whole Home and Community Care (HACC) Program in New South Wales over same period. This suggests that there were improvements in service efficiency that could be attributed at least in part to the significant improvements in levels of communication and cooperation between individuals in different services.

In addition to serving a useful purpose it is hoped that this chapter has provided a reminder that just as clients need to be cared for so do individuals and teams. In fact, caring for individual team members and the team increases our capacity to care for clients.

As one community service coordinator in a small rural community involved in the demonstration project in Tamworth observed: 'I felt very isolated before, but now it feels like I'm part of a team. It's so much easier to make case plans and to know what is going on when you can meet people and talk to them over a table.' *This is why making teams work matters!*

Finally, try this recap exercise (Box 13.2).

Box 13.2: Reassessment—Team Assessment Quiz

1 Gather the data from your initial assessment and redo the assessment using the language concepts and your understandings of this chapter.
2 You should have noticed that if you assessed your team as working well in your initial assessment, it was primarily due to the fact that the group either deliberately or inadvertently followed the processes suggested in this chapter.

NOTES

Disclaimer: This chapter represents the views of the authors, not necessarily those of the NSW Department of Ageing, Disability and Home Care.

1 Rubenstein, L. and Sadler, P. *Changing Care for Older People: Trialing New Ideas.* Social Policy Directorate Best Practice Paper No. 3. Sydney: Office on Ageing, 1994.
2 House of Representatives Standing Committee on Community Affairs. *Home But Not Alone: Report on the Home and Community Care Program.* Canberra: AGPS, 1994.
3 Department of Health, Housing and Community Services. *Efficiency and Effectiveness Review of the Home and Community Care Program.* Aged and Community Care Service Development and Evaluation Report No. 18. Canberra: AGPS, 1995.
4 Rubenstein, L. and Sadler, P. *Changing Care for Older People: Trialing New Ideas.* Social Policy Directorate Best Practice Paper No. 3. Sydney: Office on Ageing, 1994.
5 Sadler, P. and Owen, A. Directions in community care reform: a NSW example. *Australian Journal on Ageing* May 1996, 15 (2): 87–8.
6 Rubenstein, L. and Sadler, P. *Changing Care for Older People: Trialing New Ideas.* Social Policy Directorate Best Practice Paper No. 3. Sydney: Office on Ageing, 1994.
7 Fine, M. Thomson, C. and Graham, S. *Demonstration Projects in Integrated Community Care: Final Evaluation Report.* Sydney: Social Policy Research Centre, University of New South Wales, 1998.

8 Ageing and Disability Department. *Community Solutions.* Issue 4. Sydney: Ageing and Disability Department, 1998.
9 Fine, M., Thomson, C. and Graham, S. *Demonstration Projects in Integrated Community Care: Final Evaluation Report.* Sydney: Social Policy Research Centre, University of New South Wales, 1998.
10 Tuckman, B.W. Developmental sequence in small groups. *Psychological Bulletin* 1965, 63: 384–9.
11 Tuckman, B.W. and Jensen, M.A. Stages in small group development revisited. *Group and Organisation Studies* 1997, 2 (4): 419–27.
12 Tuckman, B.W. Developmental sequence in small groups. *Psychological Bulletin* 1965, 63: 384–9.
13 Tuckman, B.W. and Jensen, M.A. Stages in small group development revisited. *Group and Organisation Studies* 1997, 2 (4): 419–27.
14 Fine, M., Thomson, C. and Graham, S. *Demonstration Projects in Integrated community Care: Final Evaluation Report.* Sydney: Social Policy Research Centre, University of New South Wales, 1998.
15 Ageing and Disability Department. *Community Care Assessment in NSW: A Framework for the Future. Discussion Paper.* Sydney, 1998.

14

Working with the media

Peter Baume and Alix Magney

The kind of communication you use when getting your message to the media will be different from the kind of communication you use when you are working with individuals, organisations, and bureaucracies. Working with the media requires carefully honed communication skills. So it is worth our while, and our time, to try to understand some features of communication, so that we can then cross the gulf that seems to divide the world of journalism from so many other territories. This chapter is written from the perspective of two professionals with experience in health contexts and working with the media. Their experiences will also be easily understood by undergraduates and recent graduates.

FEATURES OF COMMUNICATING WITH THE MEDIA

Communicating with the media is a multifaceted process combining verbal and non-verbal interactions. This means that relations with the media have the potential to be complex and confusing. To help ward off these problems we will state some tips that, if followed, will make your media contact more effective. They can be applied whether you are talking with a print journalist, being interviewed for an electronic medium, or just attempting to get your message to the media at large.

Non-verbal communication

The first tip applicable to any communication medium is that the majority of communication will be non-verbal. Just as in a small group you 'cannot not communicate', so on an electronic medium, or in print, you will communicate in myriad non-verbal ways.

Journalists will have to interact personally with the person in any case. They will 'read' non-verbal communication well, often better than they will understand technical content. They are people and can interpret non-verbal signals as well as anyone else. More than that, they are specially trained in communication, and will be sensitive to a lot of cues that others may miss or consider unimportant.

Some people might try to assert that there is little non-verbal communication in print. They would be wrong. A reading of articles in any popular magazine, or in any newspaper, will reveal how often the journalist paints a picture for the reader, with descriptions of clothing, of surroundings, of food, of habits, of tone of voice, of words used, and so forth. All these are designed to communicate to the reader some things about the subject independent of the particular content, and almost all are the equivalent of non-verbal communication.

A glance at advertising also highlights non-verbal communication of messages. Again, this is common to both print and **electronic media**. While some advertisers transmit a lot of content, and may suffer in the process, others rely on more subtle messages, often delivered through non-verbal means, to get across important selling messages. For example, some products are linked by advertisers with sexual or life success, using carefully crafted environments and associations to make their messages effective. The choices of messengers, clothing, surroundings, and colleagues, are all considered carefully by advertisers, for each may give 'cues' to possible recipients of the message.

TIP: It has been estimated that two-thirds to three-quarters of all communication might be non-verbal, and to ignore such a powerful contribution to communication is just foolish.

Let us consider some of the more specific aspects of communicating with the media.

Making contact

You may wish to consider first how to let the media know that you are interested in being part of a story.

The matter may not arise if the question is one that is of high current interest to media. So, if there is a war, an epidemic, a natural disaster, or a breakdown in societal arrangements, the media may seek out recognised experts and may want to discuss aspects of the current problem with you. The journalist, a 'bridge' between the expert and a wider public, has a task to make clearer the nature of the event and some possible 'solutions'.

Many of these approaches can be anticipated, and, if you want to appear to maximum advantage, you should rehearse the likely questions and the best answers to those questions well in advance of any approach. If 'caught out' you can always arrange for a delay before meeting the journalist. This is often necessary anyhow for logistical reasons, and you should then use any intervening time to prepare for the interview.

If you are a recognised expert, however, or if you are part of a group that has expertise, it may be desirable to draw attention to what you have to offer to the story. Remember that journalists owe more to their publics than they do to you and they will not come to you unless they see an advantage to themselves or to those they serve. If you are boring them they will often not hesitate to end the contact.

CHOICES IN WRITTEN COMMUNICATIONS

Written communication is one of the best ways of getting your message to the media but not all written communication sends the same message. A media or **press release** is the way of directly notifying media outlets of your message. Articles, reports, or stories are more formal, less immediate forms of written communication. The nature of your message will determine which form of written communication to use. If it is an urgent notification or announcement of research findings, government funding, or publication of a book for example, then a release is the best method. If, however, your message does not require the urgency of a release, but more thoughtful consideration, then an article or report may better suit.

Media releases

Often contact is by media or press release. This means that the person outside journalism initiates the approach—not the journalist. Some media organisations receive hundreds of press releases each day and you will have to work to have your particular release noted and acted on, and not 'filed' forthwith in the waste bin. Adherence to certain 'rules' makes it more likely that a press release will not be ignored or rejected summarily.

First, the release should say something. The habit of some political press secretaries issuing a set number of releases each day is often counter-productive. The releases sometimes are light on news, or other significant content, and may contain a lot of rhetoric and propaganda instead. They are likely to be ignored by editors.

Second, the release should be attention grabbing. It might be printed on brightly coloured paper. It might make innovative use of space or illustrations.

Third, the release should be completely contained in one page. No recipient should have to turn over or to go to other pages. The exception to this rule is that any release could, if needed, contain an appendix, which people may or may not choose to read. But the release itself should be complete in less than one page. The preparation of such short releases is good training in any case. They force you to write with precision and focus on the key issues.

Some releases are not well written. The habit of those trained in science to write with the conclusion later in the piece, even at the end, is not the way journalists should write. For journalists, the conclusion, the finding, the *gravamen* of the story, should be stated in the first sentence if possible, and certainly in the first paragraph.

Newspaper stories are shortened if necessary to fit the space between paid advertisements. When cut, they are often cut from the bottom so that later conclusions are more likely to be lost. So, for practical reasons, many people put conclusions early. It is also often better communication, making clear early on what the piece is all about.

Radio and television stories also need to be truncated or cut to fit the time available. It is the available time that determines what appears, not often the inherent value of what is being said. Disasters may cause variations to this rule, but on most occasions time is limited and fixed.

Headlines are written by editorial staff. These are not necessarily the same people who write the story. In writing a headline, a 'spin' is often placed on the story and many people do no more than scan the headings before deciding selectively which articles they will read. So, to a certain extent, you are 'hostage' to the writers of headlines or to the introducers of programs on electronic media.

The language used in any release, or in any article should be simple and direct. Short words are better than long words. Simple ideas are to be preferred to complex ones.

TIP: To write a succinct release remember to follow the 'five Ws and how'. These should all be included in the first paragraph. Once you have reduced your message to its essence, communicating it to journalists should be relatively simple. (Chapter 12 covers the five Ws.)

Articles, reports, and stories

This section covers writing for newspapers as well as reports and stories for non-specialist audiences. The first thing to understand is that most **print media** operate commercially and their business is entertainment. If something is not entertaining, or if it is likely to lose part of their readership, it will not get coverage. Further, if it is likely to offend their advertisers, they might not have an interest in it.

Newspapers live by selling advertising, either classified advertising or display advertising. News stories exist to fill the space between the paid advertisements, and may have, as another purpose, the attraction of a specific readership, which allows the newspaper to present particular demographic characteristics of the readership to potential advertisers. Almost the same applies to the electronic media, which 'tailor' particular items to the segment of the population to which they are talking, and not to anyone else.

But why is it that academics are not generally welcomed by newspapers and other print media? Academics write dryly. They are sometimes dense. They value accuracy. They are light on adjectives and 'colour'. They value the ability to reproduce their findings. They are real children of René Descartes.

Journalists differ. Apart from writing for their editors, journalists write or speak for their publics. They use adjectives. They like colour. They are good at non-verbal communication. They like 'atmosphere'. They are not interested in turning their publics off, and they are sensitive to the reaction to what they do or say, particularly reaction from their advertisers. They value communication over anything else.

'Experts' and journalists might see the same things quite differently. For instance, each year, one large organisation gives out some media awards. It appoints, as judges, five people, two in the area of health and three journalists. One year, the votes were three to two on most awards, the journalists voting for the best story, the most felicitous communication, but with the health people voting for the best health report. It was not a case of good and bad, or of right or wrong, but it was a case of two valid, but different, ways of seeing the same events.

The journalists saw the demands of their calling, its skills, the possibilities of presentation, the craft of writing, composing, and presenting. They emphasised the process of communication. The health people were concerned with the importance of the issue, the quality of the intervention, the potential importance of the intervention to humankind, the significance of the advance, the validity of the assertions. They tended to emphasise the likely outcomes of the intervention.

TIP: Remember the media have different assumptions, different emphases, and different ways of assessing the same pieces of writing.

LIVE COMMUNICATION

Many of the skills of devising and creating a succinct, simple message are equally applicable to live communication with the media. The big differences with live communication are the immediacy and the 'liveness' of the contact. These two features introduce a new set of criteria for effective and efficient communication. We offer suggestions for live communication that will help your message be successfully delivered and eagerly received.

Live it

Often scientists, including social scientists, are boring whenever they get in front of a television camera. Routinely they are perceived as 'boffins', remote or other-worldly figures unable to communicate with the 'real' world.

It is important to note there are cultural differences between media, academe, and other people that affect how each sees the other. They just see and interpret the world differently. Just consider how differently Jim Hacker thinks from Sir Humphrey Appleby. It is recorded that a former Australian prime minister and his then public service chief sat down together to watch an episode of *Yes, Minister*. Both laughed, but at different places.

There is a mass of communication, especially relevant to electronic media, that is associated with non-verbal cues. With radio, the tone of voice is important. You should sound as you wish to be heard, cultivating an accent that does not put people off unnecessarily, and you should project a personality that is pleasant and non-threatening. With television, non-verbal communication becomes even more important. How you stand or sit, what you wear, how you are made up, how you smile, whether you look at the questioner directly, what you do with your hands, are all important. Any interviewee should consider carefully all these matters well in advance, and should understand that the viewer, who may not follow the technical argument well, will form some judgement on non-verbal communication clues, and will do so quickly. In that regard, it is worth remembering that many healers say that they can make a number of accurate deductions about people before anything has been said, on the basis of non-verbal clues alone.

The spokespeople who can follow the rules above often communicate well with a wider public. They marry science and data with the communication needs and imperatives of the media. What they do may be to the advantage of both sides.

TIP: Use Box 14.1 as a reminder for live communications.

Box 14.1: Live communication

Television

Appearance—hair, jewellery, clothing, particularly from the shoulders up
Body language—attempt to be calm, avoid gesticulation, touching, or tugging your face. Keep your hands still. Camera operators focus on fidgeting hands.
Voice—tone, accent

Radio

Voice—tone, accent, cadence
Language—keep the messages simple, direct, and jargon-free

Print

Language—keep the message to a quotable length
Photograph (if used)—be aware of appearance

Interviews

Interviews can be organised in advance with radio, television, or print journalists, or they may be impromptu encounters. Interviews can be conducted one-on-one, or you may be one of a number of panelists or guests. No matter how or when the interview takes place, preparation is the key.

Many journalists ask 'closed' questions, that is, questions that can be answered 'yes' or 'no'. Most professionals, especially those in healing professions, are taught to ask 'open' questions in which the person answering must give more expansive answers. It is often distressing to trained communicators when health professionals ask 'closed' questions.

Many journalists ask 'closed' questions, partly because they have been trained that way, sometimes because of time pressures, sometimes because they wish to put their own views on a matter. On one occasion a journalist asked one of the authors a very long 'closed' question and was nonplussed with the answer 'yes' when it came. So be ready for 'closed' questions. You may answer them as if they are 'open' or you may answer them as they stand.

Next, you should appreciate clearly how little time is available for most interviews, especially those on electronic media. This is especially so if you are hoping to be part of a news broadcast when ruthless editing is likely to occur. If you are being broadcast 'live' then there may be more freedom to put your view. But you need to establish ahead of time the 'rules of engagement' for the interview. Ask if it will it be live or pre-recorded for later editing. Some professionals tape record each interview to guard against the (unlikely) contingency that answers and questions might be transposed to give a misleading impression of what actually was said.

Many open-line radio hosts will cut off a boring or long-winded speaker, and many have as their touchstone that what is being presented must be good entertainment, almost irrespective of whether its content is good. Because entertainment is the goal, many presenters will favour 'confrontational' interviews, in which people of widely divergent views will be part of the same interview.

Which leads to the next point. Be sure, when communicating to the public, to do as is done in print and by others: put the main message up front and be sure that it comes across during the interview. The rule in all interviews, as in media releases, is that the main message should be in the first sentence if possible, and should certainly be in the first paragraph. You should use simple words if they suffice, and avoid technical jargon if at all possible. Answers should be short and precise. The habit of some professionals to keep talking almost *ad infinitum* is annoying, and likely to turn off listeners or viewers.

You should answer the question if possible. Some people do not answer questions put to them and this is noted, even by unsophisticated receivers.

It is easy for interviews to drift into allied but sufficiently different topic areas; do not be afraid to redirect the interviewer to the issues at stake. One way is to acknowledge the issue that has been raised as being an important, and associated concern, but outside the scope of what is being discussed at the moment. Naturally this redirection takes a degree of subtlety and tact.

With most interviews it is possible to formulate the likely questions and possible answers in advance. Those communicating with the media should do this.

TIP: Remember preparation is the key. The message must be simple because time is short.

TIMELINESS OF INFORMATION

News has the habit of going stale quickly. This means that the release time of your message must be carefully considered.

Stale and fresh news

News is determined not just by the content but also by its exclusivity and freshness. All forms of media like to be the first to bring 'new' news. Therefore make sure all the suitable media outlets, including local papers and trade magazines, are contacted with exactly the same information and photograph (if used) within a few hours. Information after the event is stale.

Exclusives

Sometimes, exclusivity can be used as a way of ensuring coverage in a particular medium. You may like to offer your story as an 'exclusive' to either television or a newspaper. By doing this you offer the outlet the opportunity to break the story to the public. Working out who gets the exclusive can be tricky. A friend in public relations observed that she offers exclusives to the media outlet that provides the best instrument for communication, bearing in mind that relationships can be built or broken on the back of an exclusive. It is important to note that this particularised approach can backfire if the media outlet accepts the exclusive coverage, and then doesn't air or print the story. Hence the relationship with the particular outlet or individual may influence choice.

TIP: Remember, there are no guarantees that your story will get coverage—use exclusives wisely.

Time of release

Your story competes with hundreds of other local stories and innumerable international stories. To the best of your ability find a 'good' time to release the information. Mid to late morning media conferences and media releases are ideal. It gives the journalist enough time to put together a story for the evening television news or for the following morning's print news.

The other aspect of timely release is to be aware of other news stories. It is difficult to get another opportunity once it has been released. For example, try not to release your message immediately following a local disaster. Media outlets will be concerned with covering the disaster and your message will be lost in the aftermath. As an example of timely release, Carl Scully, Minister for Transport in New South Wales, often releases stories with media conferences held on-site on Sunday. Sunday is a notoriously slow news day. This means that transport stories regularly appear on the Sunday evening television news and the Monday morning papers.

The final message about time of release is that you cannot control everything. Sometimes press releases and media conferences are well attended and receive little coverage, while at other times the opposite happens.

Communication technologies

Internet and email are some of the latest communication technologies. They provide a service both for incoming and outgoing information. Just like other forms of communication, emailed information competes for attention.

Generally speaking, media releases are mostly done via the Internet except if there is a gimmick, gift, or other attention-seeking item attached to the release. As mentioned, the essence of the message must be contained in the first paragraph. Attachments should only contain supplementary details for the story. If the journalist's attention is not grabbed by the first paragraph, it is unlikely that the attachment will be opened. With access to electronic scanning equipment photographs, too, can be emailed.

The Internet can be a way of short circuiting endless contacts between an organisation and its media. Nevertheless, use the Internet wisely for both information dissemination and information gathering.

MEDIA CONFERENCES

A media conference is an instrument of communication. A conference can be used as a special event to launch your message, whether it is a product or a service. Or it can be a news conference so that the media, as a whole, have access to you for questioning. It should be noted that media and news conferences are bigger communication events than media releases. News conferences can be organised far more quickly than a 'special event' type of conference. Nevertheless, both require keen organisation and a degree of preparation.

'Do it yourself' media conference

Working in small companies or in institutions without a public affairs department means that you may have to organise your own media conference. The following section is designed for individuals and organisations that do not have access to the expertise of internal public affairs departments. We have included a framework of details for organising a media conference with the view to launching a product or service.

We have included a timeline in Box 14.2 of what to do when and an explanation of some of the organisational details for each step. You could use it as your template.

Mailing list

A mailing list includes the names, and postal and email addresses of all journalists and special guests to be invited to the function. Use the compilation of the list to check spelling, titles, official positions, and so forth.

Media alert/Diary date

This needs to be both enticing and informative. The aim is to get journalists to note the date of your media conference in their diary as a potential story. However, take care not to give the story away in the alert. This is a flirting tactic to get them interested.

Printed invitation

This includes date, time, place, RSVP details, plus the dignitary, VIP, expert, or whoever it is who is going to make the media want to come to you. If you are

Box 14.2: Organising a media conference

Time line	What to do	Delivery
4 weeks prior	Mailing list	Begin compilation
2 weeks prior	Media alert/Diary date	Email
10 days prior	Printed invitation	By hand where possible
5 days prior	Personal follow-up	Telephone where possible
2 days prior	Name tags	By hand on the day
D-Day	Media pack	By hand to attendees, courier to others

releasing research findings, tempt the media with a snappy headline that lets only a bit of the secret out. Use personalities associated with particular areas.

Obviously, you need to tee up these details well in advance so your personality has time to schedule your event into their diary. The invitation should also include details of the function that accompanies your media conference, such as light refreshments, morning tea, or champagne cocktail.

Invitations can be outrageous, cheeky, elegant, or sophisticated. Choose something appropriate. Gimmicks, gifts, and unusual forms of delivery are all part of the mystique and fun of invitations.

Personal follow-up

The key is perseverance. Telephone contact can be hard to make, but the personal touch has amazing results. This is the time to draw attention to your event. Do not be disheartened if the journalists you speak to have yet to attend to your invitation. This is the time to sell the event and get the commitments and replies.

Name tags

Putting names to faces is one of the keys of communication so name tags are essential. Rules to follow for good name tags:

- correct spelling—this can be checked at the time they reply
- easy to read—large, legible lettering
- name of person and organisation—sometimes titles or official position also need to be included
- have spares on the day.

Media pack

A media pack includes a variety of information usually packaged in purpose-printed A4 folders that tie in with the theme of the event, invitation, and story you are selling.

Box 14.3: Contents of a media pack

- Media release for the day (newsy)
- Fact sheet—slightly different details from above
- Background sheet—to flesh out the story
- Biography on dignitary, VIP, or expert
- Photographs (if appropriate)—basic black and white shots of the thing you are launching, reporting

The media pack is handed to media attendees on the day, and couriered to those unable to attend.

TIP: Take care not to underestimate how much planning is involved.

INTERNAL PUBLIC AFFAIRS DEPARTMENT (PAD)

Large institutions often have their own public affairs department, which is comprised of a number of smaller specialist areas, such as public relations, marketing, media communications, and publications. If you work in a large organisation with a PAD, then our advice is to work with the experts. The public relations department can manage media conferences, special events, and promotion details. Allow them to advise you on media conference details: who to invite, when to hold it, what catering to provide, and what facilities will be required by each media organisation.

The media relations people will be able to contact appropriate journalists in a range of outlets. They will have up-to-date mailing lists for releases and invitations. They will be able to refine your message, and deliver it in the most appropriate and meaningful way.

Media training is essential. If it is offered in-house, attend courses. Nothing prepares you for the real thing like actually doing it, but practice and training can help overcome initial fears and allow you to concentrate on the art of communication.

PADs often have a developments section concerned with relationships with sponsors, donors, and benefactors. These specialists may be able to help you or your project become involved with potential patrons. Similarly when questions are asked by the media, 'in-house' specialists, such as you, can be called upon by the PAD to respond to media enquiries whether it be as an expert opinion or as the key spokesperson concerning information being released.

PADs are full of public relations, communications, and media consultants who work with the media all the time.

TIP: Work with the experts.

ISSUE/CRISIS MANAGEMENT

What happens when you have bad news to report? The response to crises is often via electronic media. In whichever medium you are asked to reply, you should deal with the issue quickly and decisively. So, on an electronic medium, you would have about fifteen seconds (or less) to 'put the issue to bed', while in print you would try to deal with the crisis in the first paragraph.

If you are to deal with crises quickly and effectively, every word becomes important. This is one occasion where detailed preparation rewards the presenter, whether the response is spoken or written.

Very frequently, what people are looking for is evidence that you are 'on top' of a crisis—if you give them this idea the content may be less important (although the content must still be credible).

An example of good management: in 1993 McDonald's found Legionella in one air-conditioning unit in one Sydney metropolitan outlet. In response, management swiftly shutdown all water-cooled air-conditioning units across Sydney, installed every available mobile unit and promptly held a media conference along the lines of *'We have detected legionella in one air-conditioner and because we care for our customers we have taken the following precautions, shutting down all water-cooled units, hiring mobile air-conditioners, etc'.*

An example of bad management: in 1998 Sydney Water detected Cryptospiridium in its water supply. Rather than taking the lead by managing the information disseminated to the media and public, the communication was confused and came from all sorts of areas. The saga dragged out over weeks without responsibility being taken by anybody.

Issues need not reach crisis point. Many organisations spend time planning how to deal with a crisis should it eventuate. Such plans are an invaluable asset and save on response time.

TIP: Prepare responses carefully, be concise, and be definite. It is easier said than done.

You may wish to read further about working with the media. Guides are available that have been written from the perspective of the media,[1] and public relations.[2]

NOTES

1 Macnamara, J. 1996, *How to Handle the Media*, Prentice Hall, Sydney.

2 Tymson, C. and Sherman, B. 1992, *The Australian Public Relations Manual*, Millennium Books, Sydney.

15

Writing for the profession and publishing

Catherine Berglund

As a practical guide, this chapter sets the goals for communication at a professional and peer level as well as at the client and practitioner level. Exercises to develop written communication to the level of writing professionally are included in the chapter. Information on what you would expect to find in each section of common professional paper formats is included, and how to go about submitting a paper to a journal or professional conference forum is discussed. Details of how to reference other people's work are also covered. This chapter builds on the generic issues of record keeping and written communication on patient care in earlier chapters to further examples of written communication.

STRUCTURED COMMUNICATION

The term 'structured communication' is used to describe situations in which the professional wants to send a particular message. There is consequently less interactive communication than in 'unstructured communication'. Examples of structured communication, which are routinely described in nursing texts, include written case reports, staff evaluation reports, nursing notes, and nursing care plans.

A feature of structured communication in nursing is the conscious and defined objective of the communication. Sundeen et al. list the stages of making a structured communication as:

- define and state the problem or reason for written communication
- organise thoughts on the topic
- write the report.[1]

While each stage may sound simple, they will be very difficult if the objective for the communication has not been thought through.

The same features are relevant for structured documentation and communication, which have already been covered in earlier chapters. When making notes in health records, the purpose is not only to include information on history and past progress, and current professional assessments of health, but also to indicate plans for proceeding further with care. The notes are for fellow professionals as well as the person making the note. As Elizabeth O'Brien stated in Chapter 10, the proper documentation is a team responsibility. In Chapter 11, Max Kamien discussed the skill involved in communicating in brief letter form. Insufficient or ambiguous information in referral letters or replies is not only poor practice, but could also be a danger to a patient's well-being. Full notes rarely travel with the patient, and the letters are a vital summary of what has happened in management of the patient to date.

When patients are discussed by teams at case meetings, one person usually has the responsibility of assimilating all the available information, and summarising the background and treatment process for the patient or 'case' under discussion. The reporting is assisted by peers asking questions, to seek more information. The answers hopefully complete the clinical picture of that person, and areas of uncertainty are highlighted. Discussion is encouraged so that the patient's care benefits from the team's experience. When case reports are presented in written form, the writer must keep the objective of communicating assessment to date, and highlight areas of uncertainty, without the opportunity of answering queries. In Chapter 12, Martin Van Der Weyden suggests different ways of reporting to peers.

This chapter concentrates on further examples of professional structured communication.

PATIENT EDUCATION

Patient education is an integral part of many health care professionals' duties. In nursing, teaching is conducted parallel to nursing duties. The three core duties of assessment, planning, and implementation, when applied to nursing care identify the role of the nurse. The nurse routinely assesses physical and psychosocial needs, then develops a care plan, and implements a nursing intervention. When these duties are applied to teaching, the nurse assesses the patient's learning needs, forms a teaching plan, and implements the teaching intervention.[2] Both types of duties are carried out in partnership with the patient.

The patient education can be as simple as teaching a patient about the important routines in the hospital, or it can be a program of preparation for surgery, or a combination of a physiological explanation with practical advice on movement and posture to reduce incisional pain.[3]

Written resource material

Commentary on patient education in nursing contexts often assumes that there will be patient brochures available, and possibly charts, for use in patient education and health promotion activities. Part of the professional skill is in accessing relevant quality resources for use with clients. Some professionals find a niche in helping to construct the materials as well.

Some publications are devoted to making patient education templates, **information sheets**, and educative resources available to professionals. Many explicitly allow photocopying and wide use within professional settings, and are conveniently prepared with graphics and visual explanations.[4] There is a massive effort in producing patient education materials, to enhance the understanding of specific conditions and treatment options.

The quality of these brochures is under scrutiny, as is the potential bias in the information contained in them. Some are produced by societies specific to certain illnesses, others by pharmaceutical companies, some by professional associations, some by government authorities, and some by consumer organisations. Most are freely available to the public.

Primary care settings routinely access patient education materials. Research in the USA has shown that physicians have ready stockpiles of patient information brochures. If they consider that the material is not accurate, or not complete, they do not use it. The most common practice is for clinicians to distribute a small number of materials regularly, which they consider to be of high quality and of relevance to the patient.[5] This critical assessment of the material is crucial, as the information will become part of the interaction between professional and client.

It is recommended that professionals assess each information resource before they use it. Two simple questions can prompt this assessment:

- Does the material contain the information that the patient wants?
- Does the material contain the information that the patient needs?[6]

Doak et al. suggest that understanding the patient's focus on a health concern can help in selecting or preparing materials for use in patient education. They note that materials with a health care professional focus tend to emphasise:

- Anatomy and physiology (symptoms)
  - — Necessary behaviour to maintain or improve health
  - — Facts about the disease
  - — Skills necessary to carry out health-related behaviour
  - — Frustration that patients do not do what they should
  - — Fear about malpractice.

Correspondingly, materials with a patient focus tend to emphasise:

- Why do I feel so bad?
  - — Behaviour to solve problems caused by the disease
  - — Beliefs about the disease
  - — Skills necessary to maintain a 'normal' life
  - — Frustration/fear/depression about living with the disease
  - — Fear about the future.[7]

Their advice is that those with a patient focus are more effective.

A balance of factual information, with capacity to deal with patient fears and concerns in an interactive way, may satisfy both concerns. It is routinely advised that if written information is given to patients, it should be supported with verbal teaching of the material.[8]

Quite obviously, if the patient does not understand the information in the written material provided, it will be of little use. As discussed in Chapter 8, 'Summaries and decisions', information exchange is only part of the communication interaction. Mutual understanding is also an important feature. The understanding may be best assessed on an individual basis with clients. It is more than whether the patient group, or the community from which they come, is likely to understand the material. The concern is whether that particular person reading the material has understood it.

Further, brochures are important supplements, but are not a complete service. Leaflets cannot substitute for interaction, and conversations with patients should still be viewed as essential by each health care professional. After all, a leaflet cannot identify the specific learning needs of each patient.[9] Nor can it correctly diagnose nor advise on plausible assessment or management options in health care.

In an evaluation of patient education material from a primary care setting, it was found that patients were more satisfied with their care when they received written information in a consultation with their physician than if they received

Box 15.1

Try the following exercise, either by yourself, or with a small group.
Choose a health issue or condition that you deal with in your practice. Design your own patient education information resource.

Before you start, look back through this section of the chapter, and especially at Doak et al.'s suggestions for patient education design.

Include basic information that you think your patients should know and information that your patients seem to be often interested in.

Draw a graph or include a photo to increase understanding.

Try to write so that you could share your information template with colleagues so they could use it with their patients.

Remember that all health professions rely on patient education from time to time. Patient education resource material is often used by different professions, so they should ideally be readily understood at a professional as well as lay level. You may want to test the 'fog' index of your completed piece. The formula was included in Chapter 2, 'What language?'

the same written information in the mail. The written information in that study was combined in a patient self-care book, essentially containing information on taking care of common health problems themselves. It had been written by medical professionals from many different specialties, in conjunction with professional writers.[10]

Anticipation of cultural and community needs

Groups with specific needs routinely have specifically targeted education materials designed for them.

The recognition of the interaction between concepts of health and illness and culture is vital, as was discussed in Chapter 2. The development of culturally appropriate materials is just as important as the development of lingually appropriate materials. The advice of those who have worked with community groups in health education campaigns is to first, listen to the community.[11]

Lists of resources that can be useful in multicultural communities are now often developed. The materials can be multilingual. To be successful, each language section is more than a translation of other sections. Each should deal with acceptable community interaction and belief.[12] That is why the involvement of community members in the development of materials is so important.

Professionals should also remember that just because another language is spoken, one should not assume that each patient who speaks that language can also read it.[13] Illiteracy is a fairly common phenomenon in some cultures, particularly those in which it is less accepted that a minimum of schooling is required for all.

The issue of communication has been recognised as a key factor in cultural and language barriers to health. Strategies include appropriate interpreter services, multilingual health care workers, and increasing ethnic community participation in service development.[14]

Documenting patient education

It is recommended that health care professionals document what patient education has been carried out as part of their care plan documentation. In some health care services, this is more structured and formalised, with spreadsheets predesigned for use with each client.

Dunning has reported that, in diabetes education, clinical nurse consultants are guided by the Australian Diabetes Educators Association. The association guidelines state that the documentation of education should include:

- Date and time of teaching session
  - — To whom the teaching was directed (if not the patient, why not?)
  - — Patient's and significant other's mental and health status

— Specific instructions given
— Teaching methods used
— Patient's and/or significant other's level of comprehension of the information presented
— Enhancements and/or barriers to the teaching session
— Goals that were met during the teaching session
— Evaluation of the teaching session (for example, outcome of return skills demonstration); and
— Plan for the next teaching session.[15]

These points are generic, and would be useful as guides in other clinical areas as well.

Communication to the community

Part of professional training can be to communicate patient education issues to the broader community. Students should learn how to synthesise and summarise professional knowledge, and communicate it to a given audience in an appropriate way. In a training program in writing for nurses that has been reported by Paula Broussard and Melinda Oberleitner, upper level undergraduates aim to have a piece published in a local newspaper. The topics are appropriate to what they are learning about at that time: for instance, midwifery students may write on adolescent pregnancy or breastfeeding, and their piece must be written for a reading age of twelve to fourteen years.[16]

This program uses 'writing to learn' techniques, in which writing is part of the learning process, and may also be part of an educative process for others. It is a personal and tailored process of writing, which is not removed from context.

Such practice would be advised in other undergraduate programs, particularly in an age in which health professionals are asked to adopt community and advocacy roles in addition to their traditional individual patient care roles. This extends beyond transfer of information on health topics. It is also related to communication on policy matters, and becoming part of the political debate to ensure that adequate health care systems are in place for the future. The professional is well placed to take part in the debate because of their insight into necessary resources and systems for adequate health care. This broader role is termed 'civic engagement'.[17]

WRITING FOR DECISION PROCESSES

In Chapter 8, 'Summaries and decisions', the process of exchange of information was described as part of making decisions on acceptable treatment options. Sometimes, prepared written information is used. This information may be generated by the health professional, or, like in patient education, be shared widely among colleagues or professional groups. Two types of written materials in common use in informed decision processes are information sheets and **consent forms**.

Information sheets

Patients can be supplied with written information sheets as part of an informed consent, or informed decision-making, process. The written information contributes to the information exchange that occurs before a patient decides whether to agree to a proposed therapeutic intervention. It is useful at the stage of weighing up a number of alternatives, and involves considering the information on available interventions. The purpose of that information is to contribute to the patient's understanding of:

- their health issue
- options in management or intervention
- the process of each option
- the likelihood, and gravity of risks, including 'side effects', in each option, and
- the likelihood and impact of benefits in each option.

As in any information process, care should be taken that the facts are complete, and are not misrepresented.[18]

While the basic factual information on each potential intervention, and common effects and side effects can be included in information sheets, more detailed information and remote effects and side effects are not always included.

It is crucial that there is still patient–professional interaction so that the more plausible interventions for that particular patient can be explored in greater detail, as well as individual patient concerns about each intervention. In their guidelines for medical practitioners on providing information to patients, the National Health and Medical Research Council states: *'Give written information or use diagrams, where appropriate, in addition to talking to the patient.'*[19]

Consent form

The consent form is a more specific information document. It may be used once a therapeutic intervention is proposed by a health care professional, or mutually identified by patient and professional to be most suitable. The consent form identifies where and when the procedure is proposed to be carried out. It may also indicate that a prior exchange of information has taken place, and that the patient understood this information and appreciates the possible outcomes from the procedure.

The consent form is merely one document that indicates informed decision-making has probably taken place. It provides space for signifying agreement to the process that is proposed.

PUBLISHING

Professionals occasionally find that they need to publish, either to comment on a clinical case, discuss features of the health care system, or to communicate results of research projects. One of the responsibilities of professionals is to contribute to knowledge in their field,[20] and to be part of peer discussion on professional issues.

Journals

Professional journals provide a unique opportunity for communication and discussion with colleagues. They publish a variety of contributions. The types of contributions that may be accepted are usually detailed on the inside of the cover, at least for the first journal edition for each calendar year.

Professional associations can also canvass members' views on the options for professional discussion within the association's journal pages. There is a tension between 'academic' and research-based articles, and those that reflect professional practice and the context of health care. Educational needs of members must also be met.[21]

You may wish to simply make a comment, and write a 'letter to the editor'. Letters are short comments, often making reference to an issue that has been discussed recently in that professional journal. They are commonly 500 to 1000 words in length. They present your own view on an issue, and are written in a personal way.

Short articles, or case reports, are usually no more than 1500 or 2000 words in length. They provide an opportunity to share clinical experience and insight. These reports do not usually have to be constructed as formal research reports.

For example, in a case report to the journal *Gastroenterology*, a large team of health care professionals, and colleagues with whom they discussed their cases, presented their treatment of two patients with acute pancreatitis. The patients were deidentified, of course, and named Patient A and Patient B. The background to their hospital admissions was summarised, as were results of tests done while under the team's care. This was as much as would be presented in a case report to a team meeting. The progress of the care was described, and in both, the pancreatitis was found to be due to interferon Alfa-2b. The case report was the summary and synthesis of what was surmised from the experience of treating the two patients. In presenting the cases, the usual causes of pancreatitis were reviewed, and excluded, so clinical data were compared to current accepted clinical knowledge. Extensive references to the current professional knowledge were included.[22] So, apart from an early professional communication on a clinical issue to watch out for, the case report has an educative purpose on what the state of current knowledge in the clinical area is.

The nursing journal *Nursing Times* encourages its readers to contribute their experiences. In their request for contributions, the editors specifically seek case studies because '*These provide a very effective way of highlighting facets of nursing practice*'.[23] Best practice is combined with information on individual case studies of patient care. One article, for instance, included the nurse's description of a patient and how pulse oximetry was useful as part of a patient's respiratory assessment.[24] A short graphic presentation on how to take a measurement of pulse oximetry followed this case report.[25]

Editorial-type pieces can also be written in short format. These are extended position pieces, and are usually backed by significant reading and referencing to other comments in the literature.

When writing a research article, take care to follow the format suggested by each journal. For biomedical journals, the IMRAD format is usually followed.[26] The article is constructed in the sequence shown in Box 15.2.

Box 15.2: Format of articles for research articles

Abstract

- summary of rationale and process
- key results
- main implication of research

Introduction

- purpose of article
- rationale for the study or observation
- reference to other key literature and studies

Methods

- sample under study
- process and procedures in study to yield data
- ethics guidelines followed[27]
- statistical manipulation of data

Results

- display of data
- summaries and comparisons of data

Discussion

- interpretation of results and comment
- reference to other studies and literature

Journal articles tend to be no more than 5000 words, and are often culled from more extensive research reports for the research project. More detail on preparing reports and papers for publication is available in a companion text, *Health Research*.[27] Further detail on effective styles of writing for professional journals and publishing tips is included in the next chapter.

Whatever type of contribution you wish to make to a professional journal, be warned that the number of copies, formatting, and type of submission (e.g. paper, disk, electronic) varies for each journal. You must check the 'Information for authors' before submitting your article, to guard against rejection on the sole basis of not following author instructions! You are also only able to submit your piece to one journal at a time. You may only submit it to another journal when the first journal you sent it to decides not to publish it. Journals can take a couple of months to decide on editorial pieces and letters to the editor. The process of peer review and assessment of other articles can take much longer.

Conferences

Formative comments and discussion, and preliminary research findings, can be communicated to your peers at professional conferences.

For some conferences, full papers are written and delivered didactically. The format of these papers is often like the format of an article written for a journal.

You will need to be careful with the time taken to present your paper. You will be allocated a time, which includes both presentation time and time for questions and discussion. Generally, six double-spaced pages of text correspond to fifteen minutes of verbal presentation time. Talking faster is not recommended—people need to hear and understand what you are saying! It is far better to practise speaking slowly and more clearly, and if necessary, leave out parts of your paper if you are running out of time. You may be able to revisit some of your points in question or discussion time.

If the paper is a presentation of research data, it will probably include summary data, and interpretations of the data. Graphics may be helpful in portraying the summary.

If the paper is an early reflection on clinical features seen in your practice, it is likely to include visual material, and a series of case reports. This can serve a similar purpose to bringing to peer attention clinical issues through case reports or short reports offered to journals, but with the immediacy of peer comment and discussion available as soon as you have spoken about your experiences.

You should prepare written overheads or Powerpoint (computer formatted) slides to accompany your presentation. The best advice is to always have a backup system for visual aids in place in case of technical difficulties.[28]

At many health-care-related conferences, there is an emphasis on poster presentation and small interactive discussion on the material in your poster. If

Box 15.3: Writing an abstract

Try this exercise as practise in writing an abstract:
Think of an interesting case you have dealt with recently.
In no more than 300 words, describe:

- the main features of the case
- the reasons for your interest
- what you learnt from the clinical experience.

you are constructing a poster, you will probably need to include some graphics, as well as key points in an overhead format, and a page or two of explanatory text or interpretive material.

In order to have a conference contribution accepted, you will need to prepare an abstract. An abstract is a written piece, of about 300 words. This is a brief paragraph, in plain English, explaining what your presentation will be about. It is often reproduced in the conference booklet, so it needs to be well set out and clear for all potential conference participants. Try to write it so that people who are not familiar with your field will still understand it. For research papers, the abstract includes the rationale, process used, and possibly, but not necessarily, a brief mention of the results.

Notes

Whenever you publish, you must give due credit to the work of others. Referencing is one way of doing that. Referencing is also called citation. Each time you mention a fact, opinion, or assertion that is drawn from the published work of others, you need to name the person who the fact, opinion, or assertion is attributed to, and give referencing details of where and when it was published. Referencing provides enough information for someone to find that original source of the information. There are two main styles of referencing.

Box 15.4: Format for referencing in Harvard/Chicago style

For a book,
Surname, First name, Year, Title of book, Publisher, Place of publication.
and for an article,
Surname, First name, Year, 'Title of article', Journal name, volume number and month, pp. first page–last page.

Box 15.5: Format for referencing in Vancouver style

For a book:
1. Surname, Initial. Title of book with optional italics. Place of publication: Publisher, Year.

and for an article:

2. Surname, Initial. Title of article. Journal name abbreviated in style of Index Medicus with optional italics Year; volume number: first page–last page.

The Harvard/Chicago style is associated with the social sciences. It is routinely used in many health care professions, such as nursing. Health care educators are most familiar with this system as well. The author's surname and the year of the referenced work are noted in the text, at the end of the relevant sentence. A reference list at the end of the document includes full publishing details of each source.

The Vancouver or biomedical style of referencing is that which is most commonly used in basic sciences and in medicine. Numbers, usually in superscript format, are inserted in each relevant sentence, at the closest punctuation mark. The numbers correspond to a list at the end of the document. The presentation of details is slightly different in that list. Style guides are useful to have handy as you write, so that you reference correctly.[30, 31, 32]

Experienced writers will be able to change their references to suit journal requirements as needed. If you are just beginning to write, it is prudent to decide where you hope to publish, and then write with that referencing system in mind. Full references should always be included, even in draft manuscripts. It is far more time-consuming, and far less accurate, to have to chase references again than to reference them fully as you go.

The purpose of your communication and the forum available to you to communicate your ideas determine much of how you will need to approach each writing task. Always reflect on the main objective of your written communication and make use of the available examples of professional written communication examples for similar objectives to help you in your task.

NOTES

1 Sundeen, S.J., Stuart, G.W., Rankin, E.A.D. and Cohen, S.A. *Nurse–Client Interaction: Implementing the Nursing Process.* St Louis, Missouri, Mosby-Year Book Inc, 1994, p. 141.

2 Springhouse Corporation. *How to Teach Patients.* Springhouse, Pennsylvania, 1989, p. 9.

3 Springhouse Corporation. *How to Teach Patients.* Springhouse, Pennsylvania, 1989, p. 120.
4 Springhouse Corporation. *How to Teach Patients.* Springhouse, Pennsylvania, 1989.
5 McVea, K.L.S.P., Venugopal, M., Crabtree, B.F. and Aita, V. The organization and distribution of patient education materials in family medicine practices. *The Journal of Family Practice* 2000, vol. 49, no. 4; 319–26, p. 324.
6 Lorig, K. and associates. *Patient Education: A Practical Approach* (2nd edn). Thousand Oaks, California, Sage Publications, 1996.
7 Doak, C., Leonard, D. and Lorig, K. Selecting, preparing, and using materials. Chapter 4, pp. 117–29, in K. Lorig and associates. *Patient Education: A Practical Approach* (2nd edn). Thousand Oaks, California, Sage Publications, 1996, pp. 117–29, p. 119.
8 Dunning, T. The clinical nurse consultant: Documenting diabetes education. Chapter 7, pp. 73–85, in J. Richmond (ed.) *Nursing Documentation: Writing What We Do.* Ausmed Publications, Melbourne, 1997, p. 80.
9 Elliot, K. Working with black and minority ethnic groups. Chapter 10, pp. 195–213, in P. Webb (ed.) *Health Promotion and Patient Education: A Professional's Guide.* London, Chapman & Hall, 1994, p. 198.
10 Terry, P.E. and Healey, M.L. The physician's role in educating patients: A comparison of mailed versus physician-delivered patient education. *The Journal of Family Practice* 2000; vol. 49, no. 4, pp. 314–18.
11 Elliot, K. Working with black and minority ethnic groups. Chapter 10, pp. 195–213, in P. Webb (ed.) *Health Promotion and Patient Education: A Professional's Guide.* London, Chapman & Hall, 1994, p. 198.
12 Elliot, K. Working with black and minority ethnic groups. Chapter 10, pp. 195–213, in P. Webb (ed.) *Health Promotion and Patient Education: A Professional's Guide.* London, Chapman & Hall, 1994, p. 205.
13 Elliot, K. Working with black and minority ethnic groups. Chapter 10, pp.195–213, in P. Webb (ed.) *Health Promotion and Patient Education: A Professional's Guide.* London, Chapman & Hall, 1994, p. 205.
14 National Health Strategy. *Removing Cultural and Language Barriers to Health.* National Health Strategy Issues paper no. 6, March 1993, Canberra.
15 Dunning, T. The clinical nurse consultant: documenting diabetes education. Chapter 7 pp. 73–85, in J. Richmond (ed.) *Nursing Documentation: Writing What We Do.* Ausmed Publications, Melbourne, 1997, p. 75.
16 Broussard, P.C. and Oberleitner, M.G. Writing and thinking: a process to critical understanding. *Journal of Nursing Education* 1997, vol. 36, no.7, pp. 334–6, p. 335.
17 Rothman, D.J. Medical professionalism—focusing on the real issues. *The New England Journal of Medicine* 2000; vol. 342, no. 17, pp. 1284–6, p. 1285.
18 Dix, A., Errington, M., Nicholson, K. and Powe, R. *Law for the Medical Profession in Australia* (2nd edn). Port Melbourne, Butterworth–Heinemann, 1996, p. 108.
19 National Health and Medical Research Council. *General Guidelines for Medical Practitioners on Providing Information to Patients.* Canberra, NHMRC, June 1993.

20 Berglund, C.A. *Ethics for Health Care.* Melbourne, Oxford University Press, 1998, p. 163.

21 Powell, J. [*letters*] Short and simple way forward. *Physiotherapy* 2000; vol. 86, no. 7, p. 389.

22 Eland, I.A., Rasch, M.C., Sturkenboom, M.J.C.M., Bekkering, F.C., Brouwer, J.T., Delwaide, J., Belaiche, J., Houbiers, G. and Stricker, B.H.C. Acute pancreatitis attributed to the use of interferon alfa-2b. [case reports] *Gastroenterology* 2000; vol. 119, no. 1: pp. 230–3.

23 Writing for Nursing Times. *Nursing Times* 2000; vol. 96, no. 27, p. 36.

24 Sheppard, M. Pulse oximetry: a case study. [best practice] *Nursing Times* 2000; vol. 96, no. 27, p. 42.

25 Jevon, P. and Ewens, B. Practical procedures for nurses—pulse oximetry—2. *Nursing Times* 2000; vol. 96, no. 27, p. 43.

26 International Committee of Medical Journal Editors. Uniform requirements for manuscripts submitted to biomedical journals. *New England Journal of Medicine* 1997; vol. 336, no. 4, pp. 309–15.

27 You can read more on this in Berglund, C.A. Ethics as part of research. Chapter 12, pp. 214–31, in C.A. Berglund (ed.) *Health Research.* Melbourne: Oxford University Press, 2001.

28 Berglund, C.A. (ed.) *Health Research.* Melbourne, Oxford University Press, 2001.

29 Magney, A., O'Brien, E., Traynor, V. Assistants and mentors. Chapter 11 in Berglund, C.A. (ed.) *Health Research.* Melbourne, Oxford University Press, 2001.

30 *Chicago Manual of Style: The Essential Guide for Writers, Editors and Publishers* (14th edn). Chicago and London, University of Chicago Press, 1993.

31 Huth, E.J. *Medical Style and Format: An International Manual for Authors, Editors, and Publishers.* Philadelphia, ISI Press, 1987.

32 Australian Government Publishing Service, *Style Manual for Authors, Editors and Printers* (5th edn). Canberra, AGPS, 1996.

16

Effective writing—making your words work for you

Natalie O'Dea and Deborah C. Saltman

These notes will outline the principles of writing in English for health audiences. Most health professionals do not have any training in how to write effectively for publication or scientific **critical review**. This lack of preparation becomes painfully obvious to us the first time we have to submit an assignment in one of our courses. Somehow, we struggle through the process with the expectation that our skills will improve. If not, we can console ourselves with the thought that, after the course, we will never have to write another thing for review.

However, health professionals are now confronted with the need to present information in a clear fashion to peers and reviewers on an almost daily basis. Often, we find that the interest comes from within ourselves. How many times in the course of our daily activities have we thought: 'That was a really interesting case/problem, I should write that up or make a note for reference' or 'Maybe someone else should try my method of managing'? Clearly, the development of writing skills is becoming a necessity to any health professional not only for the classical and academic reasons but also for the more clinical and personal activities of most of us.

GRAMMAR AND LANGUAGE CONCERNS

The first component of a good piece of writing is language. While there are many colloquial forms of spoken English, written English has many fixed rules. Learning the rules may not be necessary, however, using them may help make your writing easier to understand.

Writing style

Writing style, in particular the grammatical construction of sentences, is often determined when we learn our first language. A child's language forms the basis of our adult writing, despite many teachers' attempts at affecting change. For example, if your first language is German, you will be continually tempted into placing the verbs at the end of a sentence. The creation of plurals by adding an 's' is also confusing if your native language has separate words for plurals.

Language concerns

The use of appropriate words can make a piece of writing more reader-friendly. Box 16.1 provides a checklist of language hints to make your writing more readable.

Box 16.1: Language checklist

concrete	NOT	abstract
single	NOT	circumlocutory
short	NOT	long
Saxon	NOT	Romance
familiar	NOT	far-fetched

Borrowing an old school reader can be helpful as well as entertaining. You can construct your own tests of your language skills using someone else's written material. We have included a number of exercises to help you practise correct word choice. It is not just individual words that can help your audience follow your work. The way words are arranged in groups or sentences can also enhance the meaning.

Exercise 1: Concrete and abstract words
Consider the following types of words:
Concrete word: **nauseous** Abstract word: **sick**
My words meaning the same thing are:
Concrete word:______________ Abstract word: ______________

Exercise 2: Single and circumlocutory words
Consider the following types of words:
Single word: **wife/husband** Circumlocutory phrase: **consensual sexual partner of the opposite sex bound by marriage**
My words meaning the same thing are:
Single word:_____________ Circumlocutory phrase: ________

Exercise 3: Short and long words
Consider the following types of words:
Short word: **died** Long word: **deceased**
My words meaning the same thing are:

Short word:______________ Long word: ______________

Exercise 4: Saxon and Romance words
Consider the following types of words:
Saxon word: **dimpled skin** Romance word: **peau d'orange**
My words meaning the same thing are:
Saxon word:______________ Romance word: ______________

Exercise 5: Familiar and far-fetched words
Consider the following types of words
Familiar word: **lying** Far-fetched word: **confabulatory ideation**
My words meaning the same thing are:
Familiar word:______________ Far-fetched word: ______________

Exercise 6: Correct words
It is important to choose the correct word for your sentence. Find mistakes shown in the following sentences:

- The subjects were exposed to an exercise program for several hours. (3)
- GPs are finding health prevention strategies more useful. (3)

Word interchange

Quite often in English words are interchanged inappropriately. When writing scientific articles it is important to use the precise meaning for each word. The following list of words are often confused.

Ability, Capacity

Ability: the mental or physical power to do something, or the skill in doing it.
Capacity: the full amount that something can hold, contain, or receive.

Accuracy, Precision, Reproducibility

Accuracy: the degree of conformity of a measurement to the known or true value of the quantity measured.
Precision: broadly, the degree of refinement with which a measurement is made or reported.
Reproducibility: the degree to which related measurements, made under the same circumstances, can be duplicated.

Affect, Effect

Affect (verb): to act on or influence.
Effect (noun): a resultant condition.

Alternately, Alternatively
Alternately: following by turns: first one, then the other.
Alternatively: involving a choice between two or more courses of action or possibilities.

Among, Between
Among: in the midst of. 'Among' is used to express the relation of one thing to a group of many surrounding things. It is not used to express the relation of two things.
Between: expresses the relation of two or more things as individuals.

Amount, Concentration, Content, Level
Amount: the total bulk, or quantity, of that which is measured.
Concentration: the amount of a substance contained in a given amount of another substance; the strength or density of a solution.
Content: the total amount of a substance in another substance.
Level: position along a vertical access.

Can, May
Can: denotes the power, or ability, to do something.
May: refers either to possibility or to permission.

Continual, Continuous
Continual: intermittent, occurring at repeated intervals.
Continuous: uninterrupted, unbroken continuity.

Incidence, Prevalence
Incidence: number of cases developing per unit of population per unit of time.
Prevalence: number of cases existing per unit of population at a given time; more loosely, the degree to which something occurs (how widespread, how common it is).

Include, Consist of
Include: to be part of; to be made up of; at least in part; to contain.
Consist of: to be composed of.

Increase, Augment, Enhance, Improve, Speed
Increase: a general word that means to become or to make greater in some respect, such as size, quantity, number, degree, value, or intensity.
Augment: a more formal word that generally implies to increase by addition, often to increase something that is already of considerable size and amount.
Enhance: an evaluative word that means to add to something already attractive, worthy, or valuable, thus increasing its value.

Improve: to advance to a better state or quality; to make better.
Speed: to hasten.

Interval, Period
Interval: the time between two specified instants, events, or states.
Period: the time during which events or states occur.

Locate, Localise
Locate: to determine the position of something; to find its location.
Localise: to confine or fix in a particular area or part.

Mucus, Mucous
Mucus: the noun, for example 'he coughed up mucus'.
Mucous: the adjective, for example 'mucous membrane'.

Parameter, Variable, Constant
Parameter: a parameter is not fixed absolutely, as a constant is. A parameter can change. But a parameter is fixed for a given system.
Variable: a variable is a quantity that can change.
Constant: A constant is a quantity that is fixed, that is, the same wherever it is found.

Noun clusters

Where two or more words are used together as a noun, such as 'Nurse Unit Manager', it is called a noun cluster. Noun clusters can be cumbersome and unclear. Sometimes, they are tricky to use in a plural form. For example, you would write 'Nurse Unit Managers', not 'Nurses Unit Managers'. Also if there are too many descriptive words in a row it is difficult to understand the meaning. For example, 'Non-Insulin Dependent Diabetes' is a noun cluster with a particular significance to clinicians. It explains the pathophysiology of the condition and the treatment. To patients, however, the condition is important, and therefore the most important word they remember is 'Diabetes'.

Linking nouns and verbs

The abbreviated way we keep medical records can spill over into our writing. Quite often in case notes, sentences are lost. Frequently adverbs and verbs are dislodged from their accompanying nouns and adjectives. For example, 'For home visit today' could mean that the geriatric assessment team may be making an assessment visit or that the patient may be on day leave. This style of abbreviated writing may have been appropriate for private case notes, but it is no longer suitable for any document.

More commonly, the process of unhinging occurs with parts of verbs and results in an incomplete sentence. For example, words ending in 'ing' are usually part of a verb, not the complete verb. A common problem is when you start a sentence with an 'ing' word. For example, the half sentence 'Starting recording injuries soon' does not tell the reader who will be doing the recording.

Box 16.2 summarises some of the important components of sentences.

Assembling sentences into a paragraph is also an exacting process. Essentially, the first sentence of a paragraph can act as a subheading. Similarly, the last sentence of a paragraph usually provides the entry into the next paragraph. Adhering to these concepts will certainly aid in the speed reading of your work.

Box 16.2: Sentence checklist

Do all the verbs have a subject?
Are nouns, adjectives, verbs, and adverbs appropriately linked?
Are all the words ending in 'ing' attached?
Is the use of noun clusters minimal?
Are all the abbreviations appropriate?

Abbreviations and notations

Clinicians often write in abbreviated forms and use acronyms to speed up the onerous process of record keeping. Abbreviations are only useful if their meaning is clear. Generally abbreviations should be used only when there is repetition of a series of words (usually more than four times in one piece of writing), for example a noun cluster such as Nurse Unit Manager (NUM). Where an abbreviation can have two meanings it is important to make the meaning specific. For example, 'GP' could mean 'general practitioner' or 'general practice'. In a piece of writing where both terms are used it is important to make sure that only one term is replaced by the abbreviation.

There are recognised abbreviations that are accepted by most of the scientific publications. A sample of internationally agreed abbreviations is shown in Table 16.1.

Computer-assisted grammar

Modern technology and word processing is a great tool for writers who have limited skills in grammar. Computerised grammar checks are available on nearly every word processing program. They are quite good in helping you identify grammar problems. Unfortunately, as your writing skills improve, the utility of these grammar programs decreases. At best for the skilled writer, they can be

Table 16.1: Examples of symbols and abbreviations

Symbol/Abbreviation	*Definition*
AIDS	acquired immune deficiency syndrome
BMR	basal metabolic rate
BP	blood pressure
BSE	breast self-examination
CHF	congestive heart failure
COAD	chronic obstructive airways disease
COPD	chronic obstructive pulmonary disease
C-section	Caesarean section
CT (CAT)	computer tomograph (computed axial tomography)
CVA	cerebrovascular accident
CVP	central venous pressure
CXR	chest X-ray
dB	decibel
DNR	do not resuscitate
DOA	dead on arrival
DRG	diagnostic related group
DVT	deep venous thrombosis
ECG (EKG)	electrocardiogram
ECT	electroconvulsive therapy
EEG	electroencephalogram
ESR	erythrocyte sedimentation rate
GFR	glomerular filtration rate
GI	gastrointestinal
GUS	genitourinary system
GYN	gynaecology; gynaecologist
Hb	haemoglobin
HBV	hepatitis B virus
hCG	human chorionic gonadotropin
Hct	haematocrit
HPI	history of present illness
Hx	history
ICU	intensive care unit
IVF	in vitro fertilisation

Table 16.1: Examples of symbols and abbreviations *(continued)*

Symbol/Abbreviation	*Definition*
IVP	intravenous pyelogram
KUB	kidneys, ureters, bladder
LDL	low-density lipoprotein
LFT	liver function test
LH	luteinising hormone
LMP	last menstrual period
LOC	loss of consciousness
LP	lumbar puncture
MRI	magnetic resonance imaging
MS	multiple sclerosis
NSAID	nonsteroidal antiinflammatory drug
OB/GYN	obstetrician-gynaecologist; obstetrics-gynaecology
PEG	pneumoencephalogram
PET	positron emission tomography
pH	hydrogen-ion concentration
PMS	premenstrual syndrome
Rh	Rhesus
RNA	ribonucleic acid
RR	respiratory rate
Rx	prescription
TIA	transient ischaemic attack
Tx	treatment
VF	ventricular fibrillation
WBC	white blood cell; white blood count

only an aid to your own knowledge. Most often the comments are too general to be of any use. For example, many programs suggest that you change verbs out of passive voice. Most of our scientific literature is written in passive voice.

Sometimes, local idiosyncrasies can be irritating as the computer program tries to correct them. For example, my office is in the suburb of Manly. My grammar program continually reminds me that I am using a sexist term and suggests I replace 'Manly' with 'Personally'.

Grammar checks on computers these days usually include a variety of readability scales, which tell how easy it is to read your article. These scales are usually based on a complex formula that assesses the length of your words and number of words in each sentence and arrives at the level of education your reader would need to find reading your writing an easy task. Unfortunately, most scales are designed by and for US general audiences.

In health care writing, many technical terms are long and therefore do not lend themselves to easy reading, however good the writer. A way of ensuring the best compromise is to use very short sentences and explain each term clearly.

THE SCIENTIFIC FORMAT: IMRAD

Scientific writing about medicine and health is a skill that can be learned. Research articles generally follow a set of principles that not only enhance reading, but also enable comparison. Research articles should aim to answer Bradford Hill's four questions:[1]

- Why did you start?
- What did you do?
- What did you find?
- What does it all mean?

These questions are the basis of the style, which is used almost exclusively for writing up quantitative or positivist research projects. As shown in Box 16.3, this style has a fixed format.

Box 16.3: IMRAD

Introduction
Methods
Results
And
Discussion

This way of writing is called the IMRAD format. It requires a great deal of attention to detail. It is most important that such an article appears cohesive. In a scientific article, it is important that your reader believes that you knew what you were doing before you started, and that the results matched the questions asked.

Unfortunately, not all projects start or end this way. Quite often the project looks very different from where you started. It is best not to start with the Introduction. Clearly, the Introduction does describe your original thoughts about the project, however, by the time you write up the project there can be a mismatch between your original aims and the way the project evolved. There are many other reasons not to start with the Introduction. For example, if you take too long to complete the article, your literature review will be out of date. The Introduction is the part of the article you use to entice your audience and will appear irrelevant if it is not current.

Ordered writing: Methods first

It is useful to start your paper by describing your research methods. This technique is particularly helpful for new writers. The Methods section is often the most concrete part of an article. It is also the part you will be able to write about most easily. It aids clarity if you progress chronologically through the methods. You need to describe the preparation for research, the protocols used, the methods of analysis, and the process of data analysis.

The Methods section is often the easiest section to write because it is virtually a written history of how you conducted your project. It is also the most likely section to be modified or omitted in the published article if it is unclear or repetitive. In this section you must talk to your fellow researchers. Your research design must be easily read as convincingly valid, reproducible and ethical. If you are uneasy about overzealous editors, limit yourself to only the relevant facts.

The following checklist in Box 16.4 is helpful to make sure your Methods section is comprehensive.

Box 16.4: Methods checklist

Have I/we described:

The study population (where the study was conducted)?
The sampling methods?
The sample-size calculation (if relevant)?
The non-responders?

Results

The Results section follows the description of the Methods section. Results can be described in either a chronological way, or in order of importance. The discussion then can be written.

The Results section is often viewed as the most boring and unintelligible part of a research article because it is often written as a series of monotonous facts. The Results section should rather be viewed as an opportunity to express your creative self. Experiment with tables, graphs, or line drawings to describe

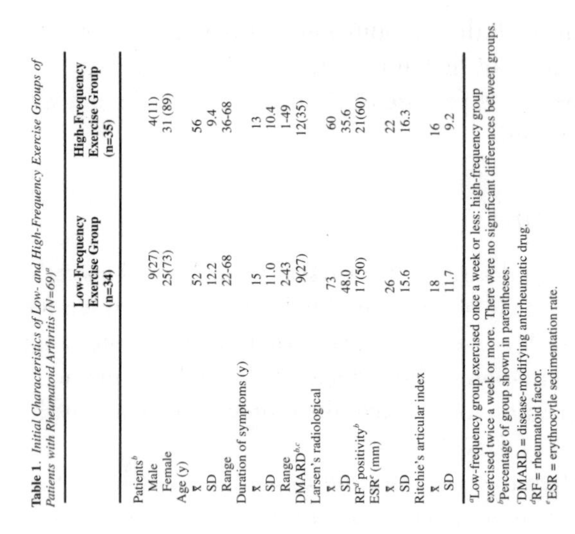

Table 1. *Initial Characteristics of Low- and High-Frequency Exercise Groups of Patients with Rheumatoid Arthritis (N=69)*[a]

	Low-Frequency Exercise Group (n=34)	High-Frequency Exercise Group (n=35)
Patients[b]		
Male	9(27)	4(11)
Female	25(73)	31 (89)
Age (y)		
x̄	52	56
SD	12.2	9.4
Range	22-68	36-68
Duration of symptoms (y)		
x̄	15	13
SD	11.0	10.4
Range	2-43	1-49
DMARD[b,c]	9(27)	12(35)
Larsen's radiological		
x̄	73	60
SD	48.0	35.6
RF[d] positivity[b]	17(50)	21(60)
ESR[e] (mm)		
x̄	26	22
SD	15.6	16.3
Ritchie's articular index		
x̄	18	16
SD	11.7	9.2

[a]Low-frequency group exercised once a week or less: high-frequency group exercised twice a week or more. There were no significant differences between groups.
[b]Percentage of group shown in parentheses.
[c]DMARD = disease-modifying antirheumatic drug.
[d]RF = rheumatoid factor.
[e]ESR = erythrocytle sedimentation rate.

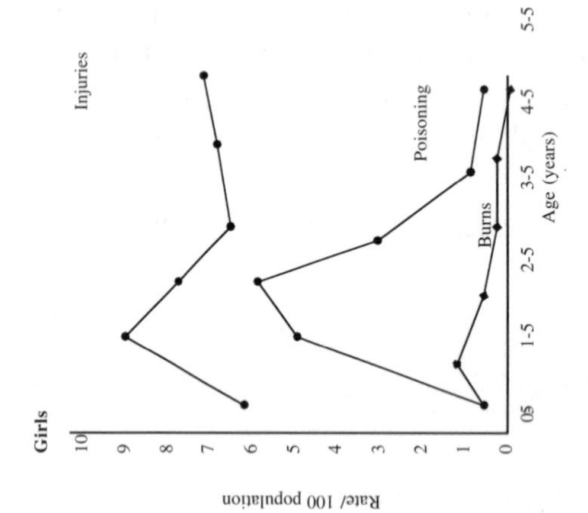

Boys
Rate/ 100 population
10 9 8 7 6 5 4 3 2 1 0
Poisoning
Burns
05 1-5 2-5 3-5 4-5 5-5
Age (years)

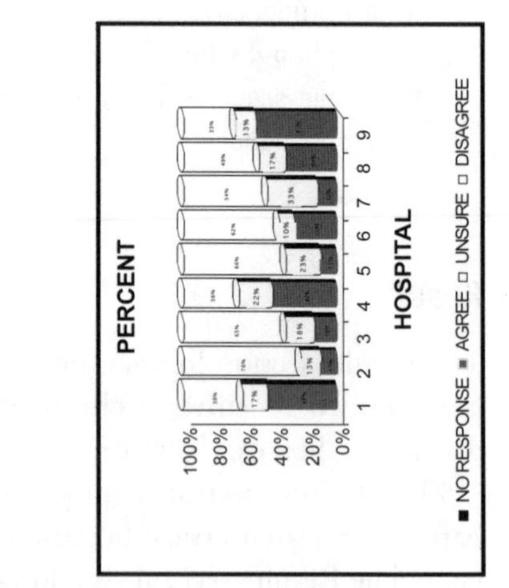

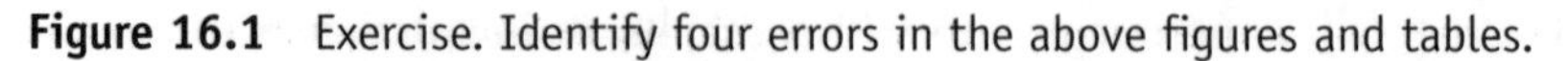

Figure 16.1 Exercise. Identify four errors in the above figures and tables.

your findings. Remember, however, the editor's knife, and limit yourself to only the relevant facts.

Try to do the exercise as shown in Figure 16.1.

Answers:

Figure 1: Average annual person-based admission rates

The main error in this table is the conversion of discrete integers into a continuous variable. By marking the rates at particular ages with circles or squares, the authors highlight the fact that this information was taken at intervals. The joining of these points makes assumptions about admission rates between the points, which cannot be substantiated from the data.

Table 1: Initial characteristics of low- and high-frequency exercise groups

There are several problems with this table:

- The definitions of low and high frequency are too broad.
- The intensity of the exercise and duration are not defined.
- Percentages are used in parenthesis for groups of subjects less than 100. This is inappropriate as it assumes that smaller groups will follow the same trend as a group of more than 100. Percentages should only be used to simplify numbers greater than 100.
- Several abbreviations used in the table are not explained, for example [-x] is not explained as the shorthand notation for the mean, nor is SD (Standard Deviation) or 'Larsen's radiological'.

The table would be far more helpful if it were turned around on its axes and the means and SDs were expressed in columns next to each other. Having the mean and SD on separate rows does not assist in understanding the normal distribution of the sample.

Figure 2: *Nurses' attitudes by hospitals*

There are several problems with this table:

- The hospitals are not identified.
- The use of three-dimensional-column histograms does not promote easy interpretation.
- The percentages are hard to read.
- There is no identification of the size of the sample nor the size of the sample at each hospital.

Box 16.5 (p. 216) contains the key points that must be covered in any Results section.

Discussion

The Discussion section should answer the research questions, explain problems with the methodology, suggest improvements, reinforce the message, and link

Box 16.5: Results checklist

Have I/we ensured that:
The study respondents are described?
The key findings are presented in the most appropriate way?
The numbers all add up?
The discussion points are not included here?

Have I/we minimised:
Repetition of key findings in text and tables?
Complicated descriptions of the analyses?

your study with other studies. The ideas should be arranged in a critical sequence or argument. The reason for the study should be restated. Evidence should be grouped into main and subsidiary points. The credibility of the evidence should be explored. Conflicting pieces of evidence are weighed up against each other in this section of an article and as with a trial, a verdict should be reached. Finally, there should be a statement about the possible implications of the findings that have been presented.

Box 16.6: Discussion checklist

Have I/we:
Explained the key findings?
Contextualised these findings to the literature?
Described the limitations of the study?
Suggested avenues for further study?

Introduction

It is now time to write the Introduction. You should progress from the known to the unknown. Explain the key words that you will be using in the article and state the final research questions or issues. Include pertinent references, including a few from the journals you will be targeting for publication. This process serves two purposes. First, it lets the journal's editors and reviewers know that this paper was written particularly for their audience. Second, it ensures that you have conducted a literature review and found that your target journal is interested in your research area. It is of little interest, for example, for the *Journal*

Box 16.7: Introduction checklist

Have I/we:
Gained reader interest by showing the importance of the study?
Contextualised the reason for the study to the literature?
Ensured that the research questions or issues posed are really the ones that I/we have answered?

of the Physiotherapy Association to publish an article on platelet aggregation and pathological investigations.

In summary, the Introduction serves three purposes: to provide a succinct review of the literature; to establish your research within a context of similar research; and to explain your motivation to conduct the research.

Summary/Structured abstract

The summary or structured abstract is the final piece of creative writing in the article. To ensure standardisation, there is an internationally recognised format for abstracts, which is reproduced below.

An abstract that conforms to this standard is called a structured abstract. Through such an abstract, the key aspects of the purpose, methods, and results of a study can be described in a regulated way. Many computerised databases, such as Medline, include structured abstracts. The eight topics to be included in a structured abstract are listed in Box 16.8. It is useful to use them as themes of sentences in the abstract.

Box 16.8: Contents of a structured abstract for scientific articles

Objective:	precise questions addressed by the article
Design:	basic intent of the study
Setting:	location of study and type of clinical care
Patients/participants:	selection and sample size of the study participants
Interventions:	exact intervention or treatment if any
Measurements and results:	outcomes of measurement and analysis
Key conclusions:	main findings
Outcome measures:	direct applications of the findings

Box 16.9: Contents of a structured abstract for review articles

Purpose:	the primary objective of conducting the review
Data sources:	a brief summary of primary sources of data
Study selection:	the type of study selected and the inclusion criteria
Data extraction:	the principles applied to extracting the data and the application of these principles
Results:	key results of data extraction and synthesis
Conclusions:	key findings and potential uses

These headings relate directly to a scientific article. When applied to a review article, the headings change. The topics for a structured abstract for a review article are explained in Box 16.9.

References

With references also, there are internationally accepted methods of citation. The two most common are the Vancouver System and the Harvard System. The former uses a process of sequential numbering of references, the latter is essentially alphabetical. These referencing systems were explained in Chapter 15.

There was a time when the quality of an article was judged by the number of references cited. This is no longer the case. Most journals will look favourably on your article if you only cite the relevant references. To minimise infuriating correspondence from irate researchers, ensure that your references are accurate and self-verified.

The Final Preparation

Notes to authors

Each scientific journal publishes at least once a year an information section for potential authors which describes the technical aspects of the journal. Your library can probably provide this for you.

Key words

In this era of the information super highway, systems of information retrieval and access have been established to facilitate the review of published works. Today, data searching on computerised databases is the most effective method of finding published works. The space for information about any article is limited on a database. This restriction makes it essential to provide information for these databases in a way that facilitates access. One method is through a structured abstract. The title of an article should also be informative. To supplement this information, most databases now include a list of key words that describe the main topic areas that are addressed in the article. Each author supplies a list of key words when they submit an article. The number of key words varies from journal to journal. The range is usually four to six. To ensure consistency of key words they are usually derived from the list of topic headings published by an appropriate database. In the world of medical scientific publishing, the largest database is Index Medicus. Most health care articles obtain their key words from the subject headings in this index. A list of major subject headings from this database is called MESH, which contains the most often used descriptors. They are published each January and July in the Index Medicus database.

The most important rule about key words is never to repeat the words of the title in the key words. It is a waste of potential resources to help your readers find your article. For example an article entitled 'Osteoporosis in Women Receiving Hormone Replacement Therapy' may have 'ageing', 'prevention', 'menopause', and 'bone density' as key words.

It is worth taking some time to designate appropriate key words, to ensure people will have access to your article in the future.

Revision

The process of revising an article is probably the most laborious task. It should never be undertaken directly after the completion of the first draft. At that time the author is too close to the work and cannot see it with a fresh perspective. It is a good idea to set aside the first draft for up to a month. The author can then review it and revise where necessary afresh. With a second draft it is useful to subject the article to several unofficial reviews. Most authors do not wait this long. Many works are subjected to some form of critique during the writing process. The purpose of the final personal review is to assess whether the article is ready for submission. The selected reviewers should mimic the journal review process. They should assess whether the article is recent, relevant, and readable. For the assessment of the first two criteria I use a peer researcher or colleague. For an opinion on the article's readability I use a 'lay' reader. Usually, I subject my work to adolescent scrutiny. A teenager has the appropriate reading age and attention span equal to my busy potential readers. If you are unable to recruit a teenager to the task, a school teacher acts as a useful substitute.

Authorship

Asher in the *Journal of the American Medical Association* has commented: 'Six people can no more write an article than six people can drive a car.'[2] Rarely are research teams so cohesive and long-standing that they can work collaboratively to write an article in concert. It usually is the responsibility of one or two members of a team to do the majority of writing. More people, however, may have contributed significantly to the work.

The International Committee of Medical Editors has laid down clear guidelines for authorship. These principles are listed in Box 16.10.

Box 16.10: Guidelines for authorship

Authorship should be based on substantial contribution to:
Conception or design
or
Analysis and interpretation of data
AND
drafting of article
or
revising it critically for important intellectual content
AND
final approval of the version to be published.

Co-authors should be decided at the onset of the project. The order of authorship, similarly, should be decided long before the writing process commences. The order may be determined by the amount of writing work done or seniority. The most senior author (in terms of status) usually goes last. In modern citation and retrieval systems only the first four authors are mentioned. For this reason many co-authors prefer to be before this cut-off point.

Where institutions or groups in different locations have collected data for a project, their contribution can be recognised in the acknowledgment if they have not been listed as authors. For example, the members of a hypothetical 'South Coast Menopause Study Group' may be individually thanked for collecting the data.

Covering letter

Each article must be sent with a covering letter to the journal. Some journals have specific requirements for the covering letter. It is useful to check the individual journal's needs. All journals, however, require all authors to sign the covering letter. This ensures that all the authors take responsibility for the article. It also means that a first author cannot include prestigious names on a paper just to enhance its chance of success. The authors are also requested to certify that the work is original and that they all have appropriate credentials to be included as authors.

Quite often the reviewing time for some publications is extremely long. If you are concerned about the length of the time to review an article, you can ask the editor in your covering letter to tell you what is the average length of time between receipt of an article and notification of acceptance or rejection. If you are unsure whether you have submitted the paper to an appropriate journal, you can ask the editor for a suitability review. This usually takes a couple of weeks. The editor will then notify you if the article is inappropriate for the journal and you can take it somewhere else. Authors are increasingly using this strategy because it means that the waiting time to reject due to inappropriate submission is reduced.

EDITORIAL REVIEW

Reviewing

Since scientific publishing began in 1665, there has been a continuous process of improving the content and format of scientific articles in response to the needs of the research community. The most significant development of the twentieth century was an increased emphasis on the review process. Probably two-thirds of biomedical journals use some form of peer review. Formal review can take place on several levels. Articles are not reviewed solely by peers, but also by other experts, for example statisticians. Editors of journals also conduct an editorial review as to the suitability of an article for a particular journal's readership. This process ensures that many methodological and contextual issues are resolved and clarified before they reach the readership.

Usually an editor asks an outside reviewer to comment on a number of features of an article. These topic areas are listed in Box 16.11.

In making these decisions the external reviewer must also consider the scientific reliability of a piece of work. Box 16.12 highlights the major points that are assessed.

Box 16.11: General questions that the external reviewer must ask

Is it original?
Is it new?
It is true?
Is it important?

Box 16.12: Criteria for assessment of scientific validity by external review

Overall design of the study:	Is the design scientifically sound?
Participants/patients studied:	Are they adequately described? Are the conditions defined?
Methods:	Are they adequately described and appropriate for this particular study?
Results:	Are they credible and relevant to the problem posed? Are they presented in an accessible manner?
Interpretation and conclusions:	Are they logically derived from the data? Is the message apparent?
References:	Are they recent and relevant? Are there any major omissions?

Editorial process

The process of waiting for a journal's editor and reviewers to decide whether to publish your work or not is painstaking and seems extraordinarily slow. However, there is a sequence of events that must occur at the journal level to process your paper.

When the paper arrives at the journal it is registered and an acknowledgment card with a reference number is sent to the corresponding author. The paper is read, usually by a journal editor. This is a screening process to reject articles that are inappropriate for the journal or so poor that they warrant immediate rejection. After the paper has been read it is sent to one or more reviewers. The responses of the reviewers are then assessed by an editorial panel or single editor and one of three decisions is made: acceptance without revision; return to author for revision based on reviewers' comments; or rejection. While the first category is certainly the most welcomed, the other two categories can signal ongoing discussions with a journal's editor. If you are asked to revise and rewrite an article, there is no guarantee that it will be published. The best hope of publication you have is to answer the reviewer's queries as carefully and exactly as possible. If you think that the comments of the referees are unreasonable, unjustified, or plain wrong, you may appeal to the editor. An appeal against a reviewer's comments only offers a sporting chance. In the *British Medical Journal*, for example, only 15 per cent of appeals are successful.

Reviewing processes

Statistics from the *British Medical Journal* indicate that 5500 articles per year are received, of which 87 per cent are rejected. One per cent are masterpieces or disaster pieces. Twenty-four per cent are unsuitable and not new material. Seventy-five per cent are peer-reviewed. Two to three weeks are allowed for the articles to be reviewed by suitably qualified people. The article is reviewed on the basis of it being scientifically correct, reliable information, and clinically important. Fifty per cent of those articles reviewed are deemed to be unsuitable. Twenty-five per cent are acceptable but only half of these are published due to the poor writing quality.

Samples of reviewers' comments and authors' responses follow:

Reviewer 1

1 'I'm not sure why they are comparing with a UK tertiary hospital population.' The comparison with the UK tertiary hospital data has been removed.
2 'As explained earlier, I am not sure what the authors are studying in this article'. This is now clarified in the revised objective and introduction. We are studying both the change in functional status and the outcomes of the cohort in comparison to the Australian norms.
3 'The Manly population improved over a period of three months ... This is not a surprising finding. Indeed this is the expected outcome in most patients.' The improvement in physical functioning after an acute admission to hospital is an expected outcome in most age groups, however, until recently there has been little research involving the elderly that follows them up post-hospitalisation and compares them to their community counterparts. This point is emphasised in the discussion.
4 'This article is very long. I found it very confusing'. The article has been shortened to a brief report and given a tighter focus.
5 'Was ethical clearance obtained?' Ethical clearance was obtained; see Methodology, page 4.

Reviewer 2

1 'Why was a sample size of 400 chosen?' Sample size: this project was conceptualised as a pilot project from which effect size was to be determined for a larger study. The researchers aimed to recruit about 400 participants due to the resources available and the expectation that these numbers would be sufficiently large to reveal variation of interest. It also represented a 10 per cent sample of all admissions for a 12 month period to the hospital in the age group under investigation.
2 'Description of the study population in terms of socio-demographic variables and the reasons for hospital admission are important as these clearly

Table 16.2: Common editing notations

Instruction	*Textual mark*	*Marginal mark*
End of correction or matter to be inserted	None	/
Insert matter	where matter is to be inserted	new matter followed by /
Delete	Strike through ~~ont~~	
Delete and close up	Above and below	
Replace	Strike /~~out out~~/ characters to be changed	through /
Leave as printed	Dotted line under matter to remain	stet
Change to italic	Underline characters to be italicised	ital
Change to bold type	Circle characters to be in bold	bold
Change to upper case	Underline characters three times to be changed	cap
Change to lower case	Circle characters to be changed	l.c.
Change to roman type	Circle characters to be changed	rom.
Wrong font (i.e. typeface); replace by letter(s) of correct typeface	Circle characters to be altered	w.f.
Substitute or insert superscript or character above the line	Circle character or where required	under character, e.g. ' or ^{3}
Substitute or insert subscript or character below the line	Circle character or where required	over character e.g. , or h
Close up, delete space between characters	Link characters	
Insert space between characters or words	Separate words	#
Reduce space between words	Vertical line between words	less # (amount of space may be indicated)

affect SF-36 scores. Shadbolt et al. should be a key reference'. The demographic make up of the Manly hospital catchment area differs from the study by Shadbolt et al., as it has a much larger proportion of Australian-born residents and in particular a very small proportion of Asian-born residents. The Manly area also has a higher population of people aged 65 and over than the Australian population. Most of the recruits to the study were Australian-born and therefore, the effect on place of birth on SF-36 scores would be minimal. Although diagnosis is related to functional status, it is well known that functional status varies even among those with the same diagnosis. For the purpose of this study, the SF-36 was used more globally. The Shadbolt reference has been incorporated into the introduction and discussion.

3 'It is still unclear as to why comparisons were made with the Leicester cohort'. The comparisons with the Leicester cohort have been removed.
4 'No clear hypothesis is set out before the statistical analyses.' As the hypothesis has been simplified, most of the statistical tests have been removed, leaving only the comparison with the Australian norms using t-tests.

Correcting proofs

If you are successful in gaining publication of your paper, the next piece of correspondence you will have from the journal is a copy of your article in printed form. This piece is called the galley proof. A 'proof' is a near-finished article that has been returned to the author for correction of any errors that occurred in the process of preparing the document for printing. Proofs are corrected in a style that is universally recognised in the publishing industry. A list of common editing notations is reproduced in Table 16.2.

If you are unsure about how to indicate a change, it is better to write out what you want in longhand rather than inventing a new notation. Usually, the journal will send you a copy of the notation used by its sub-editors. It is important to read the proof carefully for errors, especially in the headings, tables, figures, and references.

NOTES

1 Bradford Hill A.B. The reason for writing. *British Medical Journal* 1965; 2: 870.
2 Asher R. Six honest serving men for medical writers. *Journal of the American Medical Association* 1969; 208: 83–7.

Glossary

affective question
questions that relate to the feelings and attitudes of a respondent

asynchronous communication
a form of communication in which the sender and receiver do not participate in the exchange of information at the same time, e.g. sending a letter

Boolean operator
a technique used to search electronic databases. Connectors such as AND, OR, and NOT join search words and establish a logical relationship between them

clarification
an invitation to a patient to explain or enlarge upon a statement, often facilitated by saying, for example, 'Can I just make sure that I understand …?' or 'Could you explain a little more about …?'

closed question
a question that incorporates the answer in its body; a question that requires a short answer only, often beginning with 'is', 'are', 'do', or 'did'

coach
a person who provides direction and support to a learner

communication
exchange of information between at least two parties, in a process of negotiating meaning and understanding

commitment
a learner's motivation and confidence to undertake a specific task

competence
a learner's knowledge and skill when undertaking a specific task

competence in decision-making
ability to give informed consent (or dissent) to what is being considered in a specific time and context

competence in a specific skill
ability to understand and apply a specified skill at a specific time and in a designated context

consent form
document of patient agreement to accept certain health care interventions or procedures

construct validity
a measurement term referring to the degree to which an instrument is measuring the actual behaviour or quality of interest

critical pathways
multi disciplinary, standardised patient care 'pathways' based on a specific condition or treatment. They are used as care plans that identify core components of patient care as well as the day-to-day requirements to move the patient towards discharge.

critical review
in writing, the comments of an expert on the suitability of a written piece of work submitted for publication

culture
a complex set of values, beliefs, norms, customs, rules, and codes that socially and professionally define people and give them a sense of common identity

database
a defined set of information that is organised according to features, recorded, and can be searched

decision-making
process of finalising a resolution

deidentified data/deidentified information
information about an individual that has had details of the individual's identity removed so as to protect that individual's privacy in the further examination or discussion of the case

electronic database
a defined set of information that is electronically recorded and organised according to features, and can be searched using electronic search mechanisms

electronic mail (email)
a personal messaging system using computer networks

electronic media
forum for public sharing of information via electronic means, such as TV, radio, and Internet

empathy
putting yourself 'into another's shoes', using imaginative skill to attempt to understand the other person's point of view and experiences

far-fetched
unconvincing and distant

feedback
response from others in relation to a person's actions

field
used in electronic databases to designate a searchable part of a record, normally reflecting features. In a journal article database, common field examples are author, title, source, and abstract.

goal
a target endpoint, in a clinical setting, this endpoint may be set by patients and/or clinicians

GP
general practitioner; medical practitioner working in general community-based primary health care; or general practice

GP letters
letters written about patients by general practitioners, to communicate to other health care providers

handover
the process of one carer briefing the next carer responsible for a patient on past, present, and/or future health assessments and treatment expectations; the communication of a patient's health status, needs, treatments, and responses to treatments to ensure continuity of care from one carer to the next, for example from one nurse to an oncoming nurse

hands-on training
practical rather than theoretical learning

health care record
a documented account of a person's health, illness, or treatment in a hard copy or electronic form

'heartsink' patients
patients whose thick medical files, complex biopsychosocial histories, and failure to improve with treatment leave the doctor feeling overwhelmed

hypothesis
a conjecture stated in a form that will allow it to be tested and accepted or rejected

illiteracy
low level of competence in reading and/or writing in a specific language

IMRAD
biomedical reporting format for research, acronym for Introduction, Method, Results, and Discussion

infarction
a blocked artery or vein, e.g. a myocardial infarction or heart attack

information sheet
prepared and standard written information for patients on health issues and management options

informed consent
the agreement to undergo a process, when that agreement is given freely and with comprehension of relevant information

Internet
a global network of networks, all using the same communication protocols (TCP/IP) for controlling traffic

interobserver reliability
a measurement term referring to the degree to which raters agree in their ratings of a specific quality or behaviour

issue management, also termed crisis management
swift, planned action to address a current crisis or issue as played out in the media

Johari Window
a two-by-two table that illustrates four states of knowing between patient and doctor

language
a complex system of shared symbols governed by sets of rules and guidelines

libertarianism
a model of self-defined and self-determined decision-making, with some limits on decisions posing significant risk to others

literature review
a written summary and appraisal of relevant writings on a topic

locus of control
site of decision-making or power

mature minor
child of teenage and maturity of approximately fourteen years of age

meaning
results from the union of language, perceptions, and definitions of events that are also influenced by individual experiences

mentor
experienced and trusted advisor

minimal encouragers
small gestures or vocalisations that indicate attention, such as nodding, 'ah ha', and 'mm'

mutuality
a model of shared decision-making and information exchange

non-verbal language
communication of meaning without the use of words, encompassing visual, spatial, and audio cues and symbols that we send and receive

nursing care plans
documented plans of nursing care, which may be individualised or standardised. The aim of the nursing care plan is to ensure each nurse caring for the patient can see both short-term (day-to-day) care required as well as long-term planning for discharge.

obesity
a medical condition in which a person has excess body mass compared with community norms

open questions
questions that allow the respondent to give a variety of answers, which may be long or short, often beginning with 'what', 'how', 'why', 'could', or 'would'

outcome
result

paternalism
a model of benevolent care and care provider decision-making, like that of a caring father (pater) for his child

patient-centred clinical method
an approach that attaches equal importance to following the medical agenda and to understanding the meaning of the episode for the patient

patient education
partnership of a health professional and patient to reach shared learning objectives on health issues

peer
colleague

Powerpoint
computer-formatted presentation package, commonly used to create overhead projection images

press release, also termed media release
short, newsworthy written article for immediate distribution to media outlets

print media
forum for public sharing of information via paper format, such as newspapers and journals

probing questions
questions that ask the respondent to expand on initial responses

process questions
questions that ask the respondent to consider information and organise it in some way before responding

questioning
a process of request for information, whether factual or otherwise

referral
the process of one carer or health service delegating specific care responsibility to another carer or health service. In that process, communication is between one health care provider or service and another to ensure ongoing and appropriate care. For example a patient may be referred from an acute hospital to a home nursing service, or from a nurse to a physiotherapist.

reflection
the process of looking for common themes, or of examining one's own thought processes and emotional reactions to patients, with a view to increasing one's insight

role-play
the process of acting out hypothetical roles, which is used to explore situations and interactions

Romance
languages descended from Latin

Saxon
language derived from the Saxons, a Germanic tribe that conquered parts of England in the fifth and sixth centuries

sensitivity
in clinical contexts, likelihood of correctly identifying that a person is ill

Situational Leadership
a model of leadership that can be applied to a series of health care consultations

specialist
practitioner with postgraduate training in a particular branch of medicine

specialist letters
letters written about patients by specialists to communicate to other health care providers

specificity
in clinical contexts, likelihood of correctly recognising that a person does not have a particular disease

standard
a level of excellence required by a community or professional group

stop word
a common word not searchable in a database

sustainable impact
long-lasting impression

synchronous communication
a form of communication in which the sender and receiver participate in the exchange at the same time, e.g. a telephone conversation

telemedicine
the use of telecommunication technology to facilitate the exchange of health care information among geographically dispersed individuals, e.g. videoconferencing

telephony
the use of telephone lines for two-way communication between individuals who are separated by distance, but wish to communicate in real time

truncation
a technique used to search electronic databases, involving the cutting of a word at a certain point in its stem and the insertion of a symbol at that point. This process retrieves variants relating to that word.

value adding
in referral contexts, including information about clinical reasoning and management options, beyond that already known to the referring doctor or health professional

wait time

a few seconds added on to the usual period between the doctor asking a question and adding a prompt, or between the patient finishing a statement and the doctor responding. The silence created by this technique often encourages the patient to add additional information that may be of special value.

weight management

a wholistic approach to achieving a healthy weight using a combination of eating, physical activity, pharmacological, and psychological strategies

World Wide Web

a hypertext document system developed for the Internet that allows easy access to multimedia documents

Bibliography

Acute Health Division, Quality Branch, Department of Health, Victoria. Post Acute Care Program. *North Western Health Care Network Care Planning Development Project.* Department of Health Services, Victoria, 2000.

Ageing and Disability Department. *Community Care Assessment in NSW: A Framework for the Future. Discussion Paper.* Sydney, 1998.

Ageing and Disability Department. *Community Solutions.* Issue 4. Ageing and Disability Department, Sydney, 1998.

Allan, J., and Englebright, J. Patient centred documentation: An efficient use of clinical information systems. *Journal of Nursing Administration* 2000, vol. 30, no. 2, pp. 90–5.

Anderson, L.A., and Sharpe, P.A. Improving patient and provider communication: A synthesis and review of communication intervention. *Patient Education and Counseling* 1991, vol. 17, pp. 99–134.

Anderson, M.A., and Helms, L. An assessment of discharge planning models: Communication in referrals for home care. *Orthopaedic Nursing* July/August 1993, vol. 12, no. 4, pp. 41–9.

Anderson, M.A., and Helms, L.B. Extended care referral after hospital discharge. *Research in Nursing and Health* 1998, vol. 21, pp. 385–94.

Anderson, M.A., and Helms, L.B. Talking about patients: Communication and continuity of care. *Journal of Cardiovascular Nursing* 2000, vol. 14, no. 3, pp. 15–28.

Angaran, D. Telemedicine and telepharmacy: Current status and future implications. *American Journal of Health-system Pharmacy* 1999, vol. 56, no. 14, pp. 1405–26.

Anonymous. The reason for writing. *British Medical Journal* 1965, vol. 2, pp. 870–2.

Asher, R. Six honest serving men for medical writers. *Journal of the American Medical Association* 1969, vol. 208, pp. 83–7.

Australian Government Publishing Service. *Style Manual for Authors, Editors and Printers*, 5th edn. Canberra, AGPS, 1996.

Australian Medical Association. AMA Code of Ethics. *Responsibilities to Patients.* Australian Medical Association, Canberra, 1996.

Bailey, G., Hyde, L., and Morton, R. Sending a copy of the letter to the general practitioner also to the parents in a child development centre: Does it work? *Child: Care, Health and Development* 1996, vol. 22, pp. 411–19.

Balint, M. *The Doctor, His Patient and the Illness*. Pitman, London, 1964.

Beauchamp, T.L., Childress, J.F. *Principles of Biomedical Ethics*, 4th edn. Oxford University Press, New York, 1994.

Beckman, H.B., and Frankel, R.N. The effect of physician behaviour on the collection of data. *Annals of Internal Medicine* 1984, vol. 101, pp. 692–6.

Benner, P. *From Novice to Expert*. Addison-Wesley, Menlo Park, Calif., 1994.

Berglund, C.A. *Ethics for Health Care*. Oxford University Press, Melbourne, 1998.

Berglund, C.A. (ed.) *Health Research*. Oxford University Press, Melbourne, 2001.

Berglund, C.A., and Devereux, J.A. Consent to medical treatment: Children making medical decisions for others, *Australian Journal of Forensic Sciences,* 2000, vol. 32, pp. 25–36.

Bernier, C.L., and Yerkey, A.N. *Cogent Communication*. Greenwich Press, Westport, Conn., 1979.

Blanchard, K. *Situational Leadership: The Color Model.* Blanchard Training and Development, Inc., San Diego, Calif., 1995.

Blanchard, K., Zigarmi, D., and Zigarmi, P. *Situational Leadership II. Facilitator Guide.* Blanchard Training and Development Inc., San Diego, Calif., 1994.

Booth, K., Maguire, P., and Hillier, V.F. Measurement of communication skills in cancer care: Myth or reality? *Journal of Advanced Nursing* 1999, vol. 30, no. 5, pp. 1073–9.

Bowie, P., Dougall, A., Brown, R., and Marshall, D. Turnaround time of in-patient discharge letters: A simple system of audit. *Health Bulletin* 1996, vol. 54, pp. 438–40.

Bradford Hill, A.B. The reason for writing. *British Medical Journal* 1965, vol. 2, p. 870.

Brailer, D.J., and Hackett, T.S. Points (and clicks) on quality. *Hospital Health Networks* 1997, vol. 71, vol. 22, p. 32.

Branger, P.J., van't Hooft, A., van der Wouden, J.C., Moorman, P.W., and van Bemmel, J.H. Shared care for diabetes: Supporting communication between primary and secondary care. *International Journal of Medical Informatics* 1999, vol. 53, pp. 133–42.

Breen, L.M. What should I do if my patient does not speak English? *Journal of the American Medical Association* 1999, vol. 282, no. 9, p. 819.

Bridges-Webb, C., Britt, H., Miles, D.A., Neary, S., Charles, J., and Traynor, V. Morbidity and treatment in general practice in Australia 1990–1991. *Medical Journal of Australia* 1992, vol. 157 Suppl Oct 19, S22–S24.

Britt, H., Sayer, G.P., Miller, G.C., Charles, J., Scahill, S., Horn, F., Bhasale, A., and McGeechan, K. *General Practice Activity in Australia 1998–99.* AIHW Cat. no. GEP 2. Australian Institute of Health and Welfare (General Practice Series 2), Canberra, 96–99, 25 October 1999.

Broussard, P.C., and Oberleitner, M.G. Writing and thinking: A process to critical understanding, *Journal of Nursing Education*, 1997, vol. 36, no. 7, pp. 334–6.

Brown, T. Body talk. *Nursing Standard* 1997, vol. 11, no. 30, pp. 21–3.

Buchwald, D., Caralis, P.V., Gany, F., Hardt, E.J., Johnson, T.M., Muecke, M.A., and Putsch, R.W. Caring for patients in a multicultural society. *Patient Care* 1994, vol. 28, no. 11, pp. 105–10.

Buchwald, D., Caralis, P.V., Gany, F., Hardt, E.J., Muecke, M.A., and Putsch, R.W. The medical interview across cultures. *Patient Care* 1993, vol. 27, no. 7, pp. 141–51.

Bush, J.P. You can always tell a good doctor by the letters he writes. *Australian Family Physician* 1976, vol. 5, pp. 1232–5.

Buttjes, D. Mediating languages and cultures: The social and intercultural dimension restored, in Buttjes, D., and Byram, M. (eds), *Mediating Languages and Cultures: Towards an Intercultural Theory of Foreign Language Education*. Multicultural Matters, Clevedon, Somerset, UK, 1991.

Cassell, E. (1999) Diagnosing suffering: A perspective. *Annals of Internal Medicine* 1999, vol. 131, pp. 531–4.

Chicago Manual of Style: The Essential Guide for Writers, Editors and Publishers, 14th edn, University of Chicago Press, Chicago and London, 1993.

Chilton, E.E. Ensuring effective communication: The duty of health care providers to supply sign language interpreters for deaf patients. *Hastings Law Journal* 1996, vol. 47, no. 3, p. 871.

Chussil, J.T. Cultural competency in nursing. *Dermatology Nursing* 1998, vol. 10, no. 6, p. 393.

Cochrane, R.A., Singhal, H., Monypenny, I.J., Webster, D.J., Lyons, K., and Mansel, R.E. Evaluation of general practitioner referrals to a specialist breast clinic according to the UK national guidelines. *European Journal of Surgical Oncology* 1997, vol. 23, pp. 198–201.

Cohen-Cole, S.A., and Bird, J. *The Medical Interview: The Three-function Approach*. Mosby Year Book, St Louis, Missouri, 1991.

Coiera, E. *Guide to Medical Informatics, the Internet and Telemedicine*. Arnold Publishers, London, 1997.

Commonwealth Department of Health and Aged Care. *Medicare Benefits Schedule Book*. Commonwealth of Australia, Canberra, 1999.

Consumers' Health Forum. *Integrating Consumer Views about Quality in General Practice*. Australian Government Publishing Service, Canberra, 1996.

Coulehan, J. An alternative view: Listening to patients. *Lancet* 1999, vol. 354, pp. 1467–8.

Coulter, A., Entwistle, V., and Gilbert, D. Sharing decisions with patients: Is the information good enough? *British Medical Journal* 1999, vol. 318, 7179, pp. 318–22.

Cowper, D.M., and Lenton, S.W. Letter writing to parents following paediatric outpatient consultation: A survey of parent and GP views. *Child: Care, Health and Development* 1996, vol. 22, pp. 303–10.

Cox, K. *Doctor and Patient*. University of New South Wales Press, Sydney, 1999.

Davenport, S., Goldberg, D., and Millar, T. How psychiatric disorders are missed during medical consultations. *Lancet* 1987, vol. 3, pp. 439–42.

Davies, P.G., and Farmer, E.A. Teaching communication skills in small groups. *Medical Journal of Australia* 1992, vol. 156, pp. 259–60.

de Ridder, D., Depla, M., Severens, P., and Malsch, M. Beliefs on coping with illness: A consumer's perspective, *Social Science and Medicine* 1997, vol. 44, no. 5, pp. 553–9.

Deber, R.B., Kraetschmer, N., and Irvine, J. What role do patients wish to play in treatment decision making? *Archives of Internal Medicine* 1996, vol. 156, pp. 1414–20.

Department of Health, Housing and Community Services. *Efficiency and Effectiveness Review of the Home and Community Care Program.* Aged and Community Care Service Development and Evaluation Report, no. 18. AGPS, Canberra, 1995.

Department of Human Services, Victoria. *Effective Discharge Strategy. Background Paper: A Framework for Effective Discharge.* December 1998.

DiSC Dimensions of Behaviour. Carlson Learning Company, Minneapolis, 1996.

Dix, A., Errington, M., Nicholson, K., and Powe, R. *Law for the Medical Profession in Australia*, 2nd edn. Butterworth-Heinemann, Port Melbourne, 1996.

Dixon, B. Plain words please. *New Scientist* 1993, vol. 137, pp. 39–40.

Doak, C., Leonard, D., and Lorig, K. Selecting, preparing, and using materials, in K. Lorig and associates (eds), *Patient Education: A Practical Approach*, 2nd edn. Sage Publications, Thousand Oaks, Calif., 1996, pp. 117–29.

Donovan, T. (ed.). *The Falstaff Plays of William Shakespeare.* Angus & Robertson, Sydney, 1925.

Doughty, K., Cameron, K., and Garner, P. Three generations of telecare of the elderly. *Journal of Telemedicine and Telecare* 1996, vol. 2, no. 2, pp. 71–80.

Drew, N. Exclusion and confirmation: A phenomenology of patients' experiences with caregivers. *IMAGE: A Journal of Nursing Scholarship* 1986, vol. 18, no. 2, pp. 39–43.

Duerson, M.C., Romrell, L.J., and Stevens, C.B. Impacting faculty teaching and student performance: Nine years' experience with the Objective Structured Clinical Examination. *Teaching and Learning in Medicine* 2000, vol. 12, no. 4, pp. 176–82.

Dunning, T. The clinical nurse consultant: Documenting diabetes education, in Richmond, J. (ed.), *Nursing Documentation: Writing What We Do.* Ausmed Publications, Melbourne, 1997, pp. 73–85.

Eaden, J.A., Ward, B., and Mayberry, J.F. Letters should be used carefully [letter]. *British Medical Journal* 1998, vol. 316, p. 1831.

Ebden, P., Carey, O.J., Bhatt, A., and Harrison, B. (1988). The bilingual consultation. *Lancet* 1998, vol. 1, no. 1 (8581), p. 347.

Editorial. Practical procedures for nurses—Pulse oximetry—2. *Nursing Times* 2000, vol. 96, no. 27, p. 43.

Editorial. Tackling the twin faces of anorexia: Physiotherapy's role in helping sufferers correct distorted body images, *Frontline* 2000, March 15, pp. 10–11.

Editorial. Writing for Nursing Times. *Nursing Times* 2000, vol. 96, no. 27, p. 36.

Edmondstone, W.M. Cardiac chest pain: Does body language help the diagnosis? *BMJ* 1995, vol. 311, no. 7021, pp. 1660–1.

Eggland, E., and Heineman, D. *Nursing Documentation: Charting, Recording and Reporting.* J.B. Lippincott, Philadelphia, 1994.

Eland, I.A., Rasch, M.C., Sturkenboom, M.J.C.M., Bekkering, F.C., Brouwer, J.T., Delwaide, J., Belaiche, J., Houbiers, G., and Stricker, B.H.C. Acute pancreatitis attributed to the use of interferon alfa—2b [case reports]. *Gastroenterology* 2000, vol. 119, no. 1, 230–3.

Elliot, K. Working with black and minority ethnic groups, in Webb, P. (ed.), *Health Promotion and Patient Education: A Professional's Guide.* Chapman & Hall, London, 1994, pp. 195–213.

Elstein, A., Shulman, L., and Sprafka, A. *Medical Problem Solving.* Harvard University Press, Boston, 1978.

Eng, T., Maxfield, A., Patrick, K., Deering, M., Ratzan, S., and Gustafson, D. Access to health information and support: A public highway or private road? *Journal of the American Medical Association* 1998, vol. 280, no. 15, pp. 1371–5.

Evans, B.J., Stanley, R.O., Mestrovic, R., and Rose, L., Effects of communication skills training on students' diagnostic efficiency. *Medical Education* 1991, vol. 25, pp. 517–26.

Evans, B.J., Sweet, B., and Coman, G.J. Behavioural assessment of the effectiveness of a communication programme for medical students. *Medical Education* 1993, vol. 27, pp. 344–50.

Faulkner, A. ABC of palliative care: Communication with patients, families, and other professionals. *British Medical Journal 1998*, vol. 316, no. 7125, pp. 130–2.

Feinstein, A.R. An analysis of diagnostic reasoning. *Yale Journal of Biology and Medicine* 1974, vol. 46, pp. 212–32.

Ferguson, T. Health care in cyberspace: Patients lead the revolution. *Futurist* 1997, vol. 31, no. 6, p. 29.

Fine, M., Thomson, C., and Graham, S. *Demonstration Projects in Integrated Community Care: Final Evaluation Report.* Social Policy Research Centre, University of New South Wales, Sydney, 1998.

Finegan, E., Besnier, N., Blair, D., and Collins, P. *Language: Its Structure and Use*, 2nd edn. Harcourt Brace, Sydney, 1997.

Finucane, P., Myser, C., and Ticehurst, S. 'Is she fit to sign, Doctor?': Practical ethical issues in assessing the competence of elderly patients, *Medical Journal of Australia,* 1993, vol. 159, no. 6, pp. 400–3.

Fleming, M.H. The therapist with the three track mind. *American Journal of Occupational Therapy* 1991, vol. 45, no. 11, pp 1007–14.

Fox, N. A memorable patient: A communication headache. *British Medical Journal* 1999, vol. 318, no. 71186, p. 802.

Fox, T.F. *Crisis in Communication: The Functions and Future of Medical Journals.* Athlone Press, London, 1965.

Franklin, R.Y.E., and Gosling, R.U.G. Molecular configuration in sodium thymonucleate. *Nature* 1953, vol. 171, pp. 740–2.

Friedman, M., and Freidlander, G.O. *Medicine's 10 Greatest Discoveries.* Yale University Press, New Haven, Conn., 1998.

Fu, D., and Townsend, J.S. Cross-cultural dilemmas in writing: Need for transformation in teaching and learning. *College Teaching* 1998, Fall, p. 128.

Gaudet, L. Electronic referrals and data sharing: Can it work for health care and social service providers? *Journal of Case Management* 1996, vol. 5, no. 2, pp. 72–7.

George, J., and Davis, A. *States of Health: Health and Illness in Australia*, 3rd edn. Addison Wesley Longman, Melbourne, 1998.

Gilas, T., Schein, M., and Frykberg, E. A surgical Internet discussion list (Surginet): A novel venue for international communication among surgeons. *Archives of Surgery* 1998, vol. 133, no. 10, pp. 1126–30.

Girzadas, D.V. Jr, Harwood, R.C., Dearie, J., and Garrett, S. A comparison of standardised and narrative letters of recommendation. *Academic Emergency Medicine* 1998, vol. 5, pp. 1101–4.

Godbey, S.F., and George, S. Getting the facts: Doctor, doctor, gimme the news. *Prevention* 1997, vol. 49, no. 2, pp. 30–2.

Goldberg, D., and Huxley, P. *Common Mental Disorders.* Routledge, London, 1992.

Goldberg, D.P., Jenkins, L., Millar, T., and Faragher, E.B. The ability of trainee general practitioners to identify emotional distress among their patients. *Psychological Medicine* 1993, vol. 23, pp. 185–93.

Gorden, R. *Basic Interviewing Skills.* Peacock Publishers, Itasca, Ill., 1992.

Graham, P.H. Improving communications with specialists. The case of an oncology clinic. *Medical Journal of Australia* 1994, vol. 160, pp. 625–7.

Graham, P.H., and Wilson, G. Letters from the radiation oncologist: Do referring doctors give a damn? *Australian Radiology* 1998, vol. 42, pp. 222–4.

Green, L. A better way to keep in touch with patients: Electronic mail. *Medical Economics* 1996, vol. 73, p. 153.

Grimmer, K., Hedges, G., and Moss, J. Staff perceptions of discharge planning: A challenge for quality improvement. *Australian Health Review* 1999, vol. 22, no. 3, pp. 95–109.

Gunning, R. *The Technique of Clear Writing.* McGraw-Hill, New York, 1968.

Gutterman, J.U., Rosen, R.D., Butler, W.T., et al. Immunoglobulin on tumor cells and tumor-induced lymphocyte blastogenesis in human acute leukemia. *N Engl J Med* 1973, vol. 288, pp. 169–73.

Hadley, A. *Teaching Language in Context.* Heinle & Heinle, Boston, 1993.

Hamilton, W., Round, A., and Taylor, P. Dictating clinic letters in front of the patent. Letting patients see copy of consultant's letter is being studied in trial [letter]. *British Medical Journal* 1997, vol. 314, p. 1416.

Hamrick, H.J., and Garfunkel, J.M. Clinical decisions—how much analysis and how much judgement? *Journal of Paediatrics* 1991, vol. 118, p. 67.

Harden, R.M., Crosby, J.R., Davis, M.H., and Friedman, M. AMEE Guide, no. 14: Outcome-based education: Part 5—From competency to meta-competency: A model for the specification of learning outcomes. *Medical Teacher* 1999, vol. 21, no. 6, pp. 546–52.

Hargie, O., Saunders, C., and Dickson, D. *Social Skills in Interpersonal Communication*, 3rd edn. Routledge, London, 1994.

Hart, J.T. *Hypertension: Community Control of High Blood Pressure.* Radcliffe Medical Press, Oxford, 1993.

Heaven, C.M., and Maguire, P. Disclosure of concerns by hospice patients and their identification by nurses. *Palliative Medicine* 1997, vol. 11, pp. 283–90.

Hersh, W., and Hickam, D.H. How well do physicians use electronic information retrieval systems? *Journal of the American Medical Association*, vol. 280, no. 15, 1998, pp. 1347–52.

Hersh, W.R. *Information Retrieval: A Health Care Perspective.* Springer, New York, 1995.

Herxheimer, A., McPherson, A., Miller, R., Shepperd, S., Yaphe, J., and Ziebland, S. Database of patients' experiences (DIPEx): A multi-media approach to sharing experiences and information, *Lancet* 2000, vol. 355, no. 9214, pp. 1540–3.

Hobble, A., Sanka, D., Poinciana, D., and Pools, F. Guidelines in general practice. *British Medical Journal* 1998, vol. 317, pp. 862–3.

Hodge, J.A., Jacob, A., Ford, M.J., and Munro, J.F. Medical clinic referral letters. Do they say what they mean? Do they mean what they say? *Scottish Medical Journal* 1992, vol. 37, pp. 179–80.

House of Representatives Standing Committee on Community Affairs. *Home but Not Alone: Report on the Home and Community Care Program.* AGPS, Canberra, 1994.

Howie, J.G. A new look at respiratory illness in general practice. *Journal of the Royal College of General Practitioners* 1973, vol. 23, pp. 895–??.

Hudgings, D.W. The curse. *Journal of Family Practice,* 1995, vol. 41, p. 408.

Hutchinson, D. *MEDLINE for Health Professionals: How to Search PubMed on the Internet.* New Wind Publishing, Sacramento, Calif., 1998.

Huth, E.J., *Medical Style and Format: An International Manual for Authors, Editors, and Publishers,* ISI Press, Philadelphia, 1987.

Illiffe, J. Professional team: Referral responsibilities. *Lamp* 1997, vol. 54, no. 1, p. 19.

Ingelfinger, F.J. Twin bill on tumor immunity [editorial]. *New England Journal of Medicine* 1973, vol. 288, p. 211.

International Committee of Medical Journal Editors, Uniform requirements for manuscripts submitted to biomedical journals, *New England Journal of Medicine* 1997, vol. 336, no. 4, pp. 309–15.

Isaac, D.R., Gijsbers, A.J., Wyman, K.T., Martyres, R.F., and Garrow, B.A. The GP–hospital interface: Attitudes of general practitioners to tertiary teaching hospitals. *Medical Journal of Australia* 1997, vol. 166, pp. 9–12.

Ivey, A.E., and Simek-Downing, L. *Counseling and Psychotherapy: Skills, Theories and Practice.* Prentice-Hall, Englewood Cliffs, NJ, 1980.

Jacobs, L.G., and Pringle, M.A. Referral letters and replies from orthopaedic departments: Opportunities missed. *British Medical Journal* 1990, vol. 8, pp. 470–3.

Jadad, A., and Gagliardi, A. Rating health information on the Internet: Navigating to knowledge or to Babel? *Journal of the American Medical Association* 1998, vol. 279, no. 8, pp. 611–14.

Jamieson, A. Legal issues in documentation. In Richmond, J. (ed.), *Nursing Documentation: Writing What We Do.* Ausmed Publications, Melbourne, 1997, pp. 63–9.

Jenkins, R.M. Quality of general practitioner referrals to outpatient departments: Assessment by specialists and a general practitioner. *British Journal of General Practice* 1993, vol. 43, pp. 111–13.

Jenkins, S., Arroll, B., Hawken, S., and Nicholson, R. Referral letters: Are form letters better? *British Journal of General Practice* 1997, vol. 47, pp. 107–8.

Jones, D., and Gill, P. Breaking down language barriers: The NHS needs to provide accessible interpreting services for all. *British Medical Journal,* 1998, vol. 316, no. 7143, p. 1476.

Jones, N.P., Lloyd, I.C., and Kwartz, J. General practitioner referrals to an eye hospital: A standard referral form. *Journal of the Royal Society of Medicine* 1990, vol. 83, pp. 770–2.

Kamien, M. What happens when patients carry their own health summaries? *Australian Family Physician* 1988, vol. 17, pp. 359–63.

Kefalides, P.T. Illiteracy: The silent barrier to health care. *Annals of Internal Medicine,* 1999, vol. 130, no. 4, pp. 333–6.

Kennedy, J. An evaluation of non verbal handover. *Professional Nurse* March 1998, vol. 14, no. 1, p. 391–4.

Kiley, R. *Medical Information on the Internet: A Guide for Health Professionals,* 2nd edn. Churchill Livingstone, Edinburgh, New York, 1999.

King, G. Open and closed questions: The reference interview. *RQ—Reference and Adult Sciences Division* 1972, vol. 12, pp. 157–60.

Kirkman, J. Writing well. Presentation at BMJ/EASE Workshop for editors of journals. Tunbridge Wells, UK, 9–10 November 1995. (An abridged version was published in *European Science Editing* 1996, no. 57, pp. 6–7, with commentary by M. Grace, pp. 7–8.)

Knapp, M.L. *Essentials of Non Verbal Communication.* Holt, Rinehart & Winston, New York, 1980.

Kurtz, S., Silverman, J., and Draper, J. *Teaching and Learning Communication Skills in Medicine.* Radcliffe Medical Press, Abingdon, Oxon, 1998.

Kuyvenhoven, M.M., and De Melker, R.A. Referrals to specialists. An exploratory investigation of referrals by 13 general practitioners to medical and surgical departments. *Scandinavian Journal of Primary Health Care* 1990, vol. 8, pp. 53–7.

Langewitz, W.A., Eich, P., Kiss, A., and Wossmer, B. Improving communication skills: A randomized controlled behaviorally oriented intervention study for residents in internal medicine. *Psychosomatic Medicine* 1988, vol. 60, no. 3, pp. 268–73.

Lee Zoreda, M. Cross-cultural relations and pedagogy. *American Behavioral Scientist* 1997, vol. 40, no. 7, pp. 923–35.

Leopold, N., Cooper, J., and Clancy, C. Sustained partnership in primary care. *Journal of Family Care* 1996, vol. 2, pp. 129–37.

Lewars, M.D. GPs can be given copies of letters sent to patients [letter]. *British Medical Journal* 1998, vol. 316, p. 1831.

Linne, Y., and Rossner, S. What is 'obesity'? An analysis of referral letters to an obesity unit. *International Journal of Obesity and Related Metabolic Disorders* 1998, vol. 22, pp. 1231–3.

Loftus E. Leading questions and the eyewitness report. *Cognitive Psychology* 1975, vol. 7, pp. 560–72.

Lorig. K. and associates. *Patient Education: A Practical Approach*, 2nd edn. Thousand Oaks, Calif., Sage Publications, 1996.

Luft, J., and Ingham, H. The Johari Window: A graphic model of interpersonal awareness. *Proceedings of the Western Training Laboratory in Group Development.* Extension Office, University of California, Los Angeles, 1955.

Mackenzie, C. Adult spoken discourse: The influences of age and education, *International Journal of Language and Communication Discourse*, 2000, vol. 35, no. 2 pp. 269–85.

Macnamara, J. *How to Handle the Media*, Prentice Hall, Sydney, 1992.

Maguire, P. Can communication skills be taught? *British Journal of Hospital Medicine* 1990, vol. 43, pp. 215–16.

Maguire, P. Breaking bad news. *European Journal of Surgical Oncology* 1998, vol. 24, pp. 188–91.

Maguire, P., Faulkner, A., Booth, K., Elliott, C., and Hillier, V. Helping cancer patients disclose their concerns. *European Journal of Cancer* 1996, vol. 32, pp. 78–81.

Maguire, P., Roe, P., Goldberg, D., Jones, S., Hyde, C., and O'Dowd, T. The value of feedback in teaching interviewing skills to medical students. *Psychological Medicine* 1978, vol. 8, pp. 695–704.

Maher, L. Motivational interviewing: What, when, and why? *Patient Care* 1998, vol. 32, no. 14, p. 55.

Marinker, M., and Peckham, M. *Clinical Futures.* BMJ Books, British Medical Association, London, 1998.

Marsh, S.H., and Archer, T.J. Accuracy of general practitioner referrals to a breast clinic. *Annals of the Royal College of Surgeons England* 1996, vol. 78, pp. 203–5.

Marston, W.M. *Emotions of Normal People.* First published 1928, Kegan Paul, London. Reprinted 1989, Lyster, Ormskirk, Lancs.

Marteau, T.M., Humphrey, C., Matoon, G., Kidd, J., Lloyd, M., and Horder, J. Factors influencing the communication skills of first-year clinical medical students. *Medical Education* 1991, vol. 25, pp. 127–34.

Marvel, M.K., Epstein, R.M., Flowers, K., and Beckman, H.B. Soliciting the patient's agenda: Have we improved? *Journal of the American Medical Association* 1999, vol. 281, pp. 283–7.

Mathers, N., Jones, N., and Hannay, D. Heartsink patients: A study of their general practitioners. *British Journal of General Practice* 1995, vol. 45, pp. 293–6.

Mathur, R., Clark, R.A., Dhillon, D.P., Winter, J.H., and Lipworth, B.J. A repeat audit of hospital discharge letters in patients admitted with acute asthma. *Scottish Medical Journal* 1997, vol. 42, pp. 19–21.

McConnell, D., Butow, P.N., and Tattersall, M.H. Improving the letters we write: An exploration of doctor–doctor communication in cancer care. *British Journal of Cancer* 1999, vol. 80, pp. 427–37.

McGinley, S., Baus, E., Gyza, K., Johnson, K., Lipton, S., Magee, M., Moore, F., and Wojtyak, D. Multidiscplinary discharge planning: Developing a process. *Nursing Management* 1996, vol. 27, no. 10, pp. 55, 57–60.

McGuire, S., Gerber, D., and Clemen-Stone, S. Meeting the diverse needs of clients in the community: Effective use of the referral process. *Nursing Outlook* 1996, vol. 44, no. 5, pp. 218–22.

McKenna, L. Improving the nursing handover report. *Professional Nurse* June 1997, vol. 12, no. 9, pp. 637–9.

McKenna, L., and Walsh, K. Changing handover practices: One private hospital's experiences. *International Journal of Nursing Practice* 1997, vol. 3, pp. 128–32.

McVea, K.L.S.P., Venugopal, M., Crabtree, B.F., and Aita, V. The organization and distribution of patient education materials in family medicine practices. *Journal of Family Practice* 2000, vol. 49, no. 4, pp. 319–26.

McWhinney, I. *A Textbook of Family Medicine.* Oxford University Press, New York, 1989.

Metz, G. Training needed in referring writing. *Australian Doctor* 1989, 15 November, p. 52.

Mill, J.S. On liberty [1859], in J.S. Mill, *Three Essays* [1912], Oxford University Press, London, 1975.

Miller, C. Ensuring continuing care: Styles and efficiency of the handover process. *Australian Journal of Advanced Nursing* 1998, vol. 16, no. 1, pp. 23–7.

Mohan, T., McGregor, H., Saunders, S., and Archee, R. *Communicating! Theory and Practice,* 4th edn, Harcourt Brace, Sydney, 1997.

Montalto, M. Letters to go: General practitioners' referral letters to an accident and emergency department. *Medical Journal of Australia* 1991, vol. 155, pp. 374–7.

Moorhouse C. Is written documentation essential to good nursing practice? *Nursing Documentation: A Symposium to Address Emerging Concerns.* Papers from the symposium held at the Royal Women's Hospital, Melbourne, 22 September 1995.

Murtagh, J.E. A safe diagnostic strategy in general practice. *General Practice*, 2nd edn. McGraw-Hill, Sydney, 1998.

Myers, K.A., Kealy, E.J., Dojeiji, S., and Norman, G.R. Development of a rating scale to evaluate written communication skills of students. *Academic Medicine* 1999, vol. 74, no. 5, pp. 612–13.

Naish, J., Brown, J., and Denton, B., Intercultural consultations: Investigation of factors that deter non-English-speaking women from attending their general practitioners for cervical screening. *British Medical Journal 1994*, vol. 309, no. 6962, pp. 1126–8.

National Health and Medical Research Council. *General Guidelines for Medical Practitioners on Providing Information to Patients.* NHMRC, Canberra, June 1993.

National Health Strategy. *Removing Cultural and Language Barriers to Health.* National Health Strategy. Issues paper, no. 6, March 1993, Canberra.

New South Wales Government. *Report of the New South Wales Health Council: A Better Health System for New South Wales*, Sydney, 2000.

New South Wales Health Department. *Principles for Creation, Management, Storage and Disposal of Health Care Records.* Circular No 98/59, 1998.

Newton, J., Eccles, M., and Hutchinson, A. Communication between general practitioners and consultants: What should their letters contain? *British Medical Journal* 1992, vol. 304, pp. 821–4.

Newton, J., Hutchinson, A., Hayes, V., McColl, E., Mackee, L., and Holland, C. Do clinicians tell each other enough? An analysis of referral communications in two specialities. *Family Practice* 1994, 11, pp. 15–20.

Northouse, L.L., and Northouse, P.G. *Health Communication: Strategies for Health Professionals,* Appleton & Lange, Stamford, Conn., 1998.

Nyman, K. WA tackles the 'interface'. *Australian Family Physician* 1990, 19, 647–8.

O'Donnell, M. Evidence-based illiteracy: Time to rescue the literature. *Lancet* 2000, vol. 355, pp. 489–91.

O'Dowd, T.C. Five years of heartsink patients in general practice. *British Journal of Medicine* 1988, vol. 297, pp. 528–30.

O'Hara, E.M., and Zhan, L. Cultural and pharmacological considerations when caring for Chinese elders. *Journal of Gerontological Nursing* 1994, vol. 20, no. 10, pp. 11–16.

Orwell, G. *Politics and the English: Inside the Whale and Other Essays.* Penguin, London, 1957.

Page, C. Looking to the future: Critical pathways in Richmond, J. (ed.), *Nursing Documentation: Writing What We Do.* Ausmed Publications, Melbourne, 1997, pp. 87–99.

Pallen, M. Guide to the Internet: Electronic mail. *British Medical Journal 1995*, vol. 311, no. 7018, pp. 1487–90.

Parker, J. Handovers in a changing health care climate. *Australian Nursing Journal* 1996, vol. 4, no. 5, pp. 22–6.

Parker, J., Gardner, G., and Wiltshire, J. Handover: The collective narrative of nursing practice. *Australian Journal of Advanced Nursing* May 1992, vol. 9, no. 3, pp. 31–7.

Peterson, A.B., and Hall, T. Nursing challenge: Caring for a patient with complex, multiple complications. *Heart and Lung: The Journal of Acute and Critical Care*, 1999, vol. 28, no. 5, pp. 373–6.

Phelan, M., and Parkman, S. How to do it: Work with an interpreter. *British Medical Journal* 1995, vol. 311, no. 7004, pp. 555–7.

Platt, F.W. I hope I answered your questions all right. *Patient Care* 1994, vol. 28, no. 19, p. 88.

Powell, J. Short and simple way forward [letter]. *Physiotherapy* 2000, vol. 86, no. 7, p. 389.

Prince, D., and Nelson, M. Teaching Spanish to emergency medicine residents. *Academy of Emergency Medicine* 1995, vol. 2, pp. 32–7.

Pringle, R. *Sex and Medicine: Gender, Power and Authority in the Medical Profession.* Cambridge University Press, Melbourne, 1998.

Prouse, M. A study of the use of tape recorded handovers. *Nursing Times* 1995, vol. 91, no. 49, pp. 40–1.

Ptacek, J.T., and Eberhardt, T.L. Breaking bad news: A review of the literature. *Journal of the American Medical Association* 1996, vol. 276, no. 6, pp. 496–502.

Quill, T.E., and Brody, H. Physician recommendations and patient autonomy: Finding a balance between physician power and patient choice. *Annals of Internal Medicine*, 1996, vol. 125, no. 9, pp. 763–9.

Rafuse, J. Multicultural medicine: 'Dealing with a population you weren't quite prepared for'. *Canadian Medical Association Journal*, 1993, vol. 148, no. 2, pp. 282–5.

Rapoport, M.J., Leonov, Y., and Leibowitz, A. Body language in the emergency room. *Lancet*, 1995, vol. 345, no. 8956, p. 1060.

Ray, S., Archbold, R.A., Preston, S., Ranjadayalan, K., Suliman, A., and Timmis, A.D. Computer-generated correspondence for patients attending an open-access chest pain clinic. *Journal of the Royal College of Physicians London* 1998, vol. 32, pp. 420–1.

Reents, S. *Impacts of the Internet on the Doctor–Patient Relationship: The Rise of the Internet Health Consumer*, Cyberdialogue, 1999. <http://www.cyberdialogue.com>

Rieman, D. Noncaring and caring in the clinical setting: Patients' descriptions. *Topics in Clinical Nursing* 1986, vol. 8, no. 2, pp. 30–6.

Rodriquez, M.J., Martinez, A., and Dopico, A. A home telecare management system. *Journal of Telemedicine and Telecare* 1995, vol. 1, no. 2, pp. 86–94.

Roter, D.L., and Hall, J.A. *Doctors Talking with Patients, Patients Talking with Doctors.* Auburn House, Westport, Conn., 1992.

Rothman, D.J. Medical professionalism: Focusing on the real issues. *New England Journal of Medicine* 2000, vol. 342, no. 17, pp. 1284–6.

Royal Australian College of General Practitioners Training Program Curriculum, 2nd edn. RACGP Training Program, Melbourne, 1999, 3–9. (Paget, N., Director of Education, Royal Australian College of Physicians, personal communication, 7 October 1999.)

Rubenstein, L., and Sadler, P. *Changing Care for Older People: Trialling New Ideas.* Social Policy Directorate Best Practice Paper, no. 3. Office on Ageing, Sydney, 1994.

Ryer, J.C. *HealthNet: Your Essential Resource for the Most Up-to-date Medical Information Online.* Wiley, New York, 1997.

Sackett, D.L., Haynes, R.B., and Tugwell, P. *Clinical Epidemiology: A Basic Science for Clinical Medicine.* Little, Brown, Boston, 1985.

Sadler, P., and Owen, A. Directions in community care reform: A NSW example. *Australian Journal on Ageing* May 1996, vol. 15, no. 2, pp. 87–8.

Saltman, D.C., and O'Dea, N.A. General practice consultations: Quality time? *Medical Journal of Australia* 1999, vol. 171, p. 76.

San Jose Hospital Family Practice Residency Program [SJHFPRP] (1994). Five vignettes of cross-cultural care. *Patient Care* 1994, vol. 28, no. 11, pp. 120–3.

Schnyder, U., Feld, C., Leuthold, A., and Buddeberg, C. Reference to psychiatric consultation in the discharge letter of general hospital inpatients. *International Journal of Psychiatry in Medicine* 1997, vol. 27, pp. 391–402.

Schön, D.A. *Educating the Reflective Practitioner: Toward a New Design for Teaching and Learning in the Professions.* Jossey-Bass, San Francisco, 1987.

Schulz-Robinson, S. *A Political Imperative: Make Nurses' Work Visible by Documentation.* In Richmond, J. (ed.), *Nursing Documentation: Writing What We Do.* Ausmed Publications, Melbourne, 1997.

Schumacher, E.F. *Guide to the Perplexed.* Harper & Rowe, New York, 1977.

Seifert, P.C. Communication—Speaking, surfing, and smiling. *Association of Operating Room Nurses Journal* 1999, vol. 70, no. 4, pp. 558, 561.

Sheppard, M. Pulse oximetry: A case study [best practice]. *Nursing Times* 2000, vol. 96, no. 27, p. 42.

Silverman, D. *Communication and Medical Practice: Social Relations in the Clinic.* Sage Publications, London, 1987.

Silverman, J., Kurtz, S., and Draper J. *Skills for Communicating with Patients.* Radcliffe Medical Press, Oxon, 1998.

Skelton, J.R., and Hobbs, F.D.R. Concordancing: Use of language-based research in medical communication. *Lancet* 1999, vol. 353, no. 91147, pp. 108–11.

Skold, P. The key to success: The role of local government in the organization of smallpox vaccination in Sweden, *Medical History*, 2000, vol. 45, pp. 201–26.

Smith, R.C., and Hoppe, R.B. The patient's story: Integrating the patient- and physician-centered approaches to interviewing. *Annals of Internal Medicine*, 1991, vol. 115, pp. 470–7.

Spielberg, A. On call and online: Sociohistorical, legal and ethical implications of email for the patient–physician relationship, *Journal of the American Medical Association* 1998, vol. 280, no. 15, pp. 1353–9.

Springhouse Corporation. *How to Teach Patients.* Springhouse, Penn., 1989.

Stanberry, B. Telemedicine: Barriers and opportunities in the 21st century. *Journal of Internal Medicine* 2000, vol. 247, no. 6, pp. 615–28.

Stewart, M., Brown, J.B., and Weston, W.W., McWhinney, I.R., McWilliam, C.L., Freeman, T.R. *Patient Centered Medicine.* Sage, Thousand Oaks, Calif., 1995.

Stewart, M., and Roter, D. (eds) *Communicating with Medical Patients.* Sage Publications, Newbury Park, Calif., 1989.

Stewart, M.A. Effective physician–patient communication and health outcomes: A review. *Canadian Medical Association Journal* 1995, vol. 152, pp. 1423–33.

Streiffer, R.H., and Nagle, J.P. Patient education in our offices, *Journal of Family Practice* 2000, vol. 49, no. 4, pp. 327–8.

Suchman, A.L., Markakis, K., Beckman, H.B., and Frankel, R. A model of empathic communication in the medical interview. *Journal of the American Medical Association* 1997, vol. 277, pp. 678–82.

Sundeen, S.J., Stuart, G.W., Rankin, E.A.D., and Cohen, S.A. *Nurse–Client Interaction: Implementing the Nursing Process.* Mosby-Year Book, St Louis, Missouri, 1994.

Surbone, A., and Zwitter, M. (eds). Communication with the cancer patient: Information and truth, *Annals of the New York Academy of Sciences* 1997, vol. 809, New York Academy of Sciences, New York.

Tattersall, M.H.N., Griffin, A., Dunn, S.M., Monaghan, H., Scatchard, K., and Butow, P.N. Writing to referring doctors after a new patient consultation: What is wanted and what is contained in letters from one medical oncologist. *Australian and New Zealand Journal of Medicine* 1995, vol. 25, pp. 479–82.

Taylor, K. Legal issues for nurses: Defensive nursing practice. *Lamp* 1997, vol. 54, no. 4, pp. 12–13.

Terry, P.E., and Healey, M.L., The physician's role in educating patients: A comparison of mailed versus physician-delivered patient education. *Journal of Family Practice* 2000, vol. 49, no. 4, pp. 314–18.

Trentholm, S., and Jensen, A. *Interpersonal Communication*, 2nd edn. Wadsworth, Belmont, Calif., 1992.

Tuckett, D. *Meetings Between Experts: An Approach to Sharing Ideas in Medical Consultations.* Tavistock, New York, 1985.

Tuckman, B.W. Developmental sequence in small groups. *Psychological Bulletin* 1965, vol. 63, pp. 384–9.

Tuckman, B.W., and Jensen, M.A. Stages in small group development revisited. *Group and Organisation Studies* 1997, vol. 2, no. 4, pp. 419–27.

Tymson, C., and Sherman, B. *The Australian Public Relations Manual*, Millennium Books, Sydney, 1992.

Usherwood, T. Subjective and behavioural evaluation of the teaching of patient interview skills. *Medical Education* 1993, 27, pp. 41–7.

Vaillant, G.C., and Sobowale, N. Some psychological vulnerabilities of physicians: A review. *Comprehensive Psychiatry* 1972, vol. 15, pp. 519–30.

Van Ess Coeling, H., and Cukr, L. Communication styles that promote perceptions of collaboration, quality and nurse satisfaction. *Journal of Nursing Care Quality* 2000, vol. 14, no. 2, pp. 63–74.

van Walraven, C., Laupacis, A., Seth, R., and Wells, G. Dictated versus database-generated discharge summaries: A randomized clinical trial. *Canadian Medical Association Journal* 1999, vol. 160, pp. 345–6.

Victorian Centre for Ambulatory Care Innovation. *Charter for Change: VCACI Mission.* Department of Health Services, Prahran, Vic., 2000.

Wallet, R.R. Tomorrow's challenges and opportunities. *Mayo Clinic Proceedings* 2000, vol. 75, pp. 981–2.

Ward, P., and Carvell, J. GPs' management of acute back pain. Referral letters are inadequate [letter]. *British Medical Journal* 1996, vol. 312, p. 1481.

Wass, A.R., and Illingworth, R.N. What information do general practitioners want about accident and emergency patients? *Journal of Accident and Emergency Medicine* 1996, 13, pp. 406–8.

Watson, J.O. *The Double Helix: A Personal Account of the Discovery of the Structure of DNA.* Penguin, London, 1968.

Watson, J.O., and Crick, O.H. A structure for deoxyribose nucleic acid. *Nature* 1953, vol. 171, pp. 737–8.

Webster, J. Practitioner-centred research: An evaluation of the implementation of the bedside hand-over. *Journal of Advanced Nursing.* 1999, vol. 30, no. 6, pp. 1375–82.

Weinger, M.B., and England, C.E., Ergonomic and human factors affecting anesthetic vigilance and monitoring performance in the operating room environment. *Anesthesiology* 1990, vol. 73, p. 995.

Welborn, T. Inadequate referral letters. *GP—Western Australian General Practitioners Magazine* 1999, July, p. 24.

Westerman, R.F., Hull, F.M., Bezemer, P.D., and Gort, G. A study of communication between general practitioners and specialists. *British Journal of General Practice* 1990, vol. 40, pp. 445–9.

Weston, W.W., and Lipkin, M., Doctors learning communication skills: Developmental issues. In Stewart, M., and Roter, B. (eds), *Communicating with Medical Patients.* Sage Publishers, Newbury Park, Calif., 1989, pp. 43–57.

Wilkins, M.H.F., Stokes, A.R., and Wilson, H.R. Molecular structure of deoxypentose nucleic acids. *Nature* 1953, vol. 171, pp. 738–40.

Williams, M.V., Parker, R.M., Baker, D.W., Parikh, N.S., Pitkin, K., Coates, W.C., and Nurss, J.R. Inadequate functional health literacy among patients at two public hospitals. *Journal of the American Medical Association* 1995, vol. 274, no. 21, pp. 1677–82.

Wilson, S., and Billones, H. The Filipino elder: Implications for nursing practice. *Journal of Gerontological Nursing* 1994, vol. 20, no. 8, pp. 31–6.

Winker, M., Flanagin, A., Chi-Lum, B., White, J., Andrews, K., Kennett, R., DeAngelis, C., and Musacchio, R., Guidelines for medical and health information sites on the Internet: Principles governing AMA web sites, *Journal of the American Medical Association* 2000, 283 (12) March 22/29, pp. 1600–6.

Woloshin, S., Bickell, N.A., Schwartz, L.M., Gany, F., and Welch, H.G. Language barriers in medicine in the United States. *Journal of the American Medical Association* 1995, vol. 273, no. 9, pp. 724–8.

Wood, S.M. (ed.) *Health Care Resources on the Internet: A Guide for Librarians and Health Care Consumers.* Haworth Information Press, New York, 1999.

Wright, S., Bowkett, J., and Bray, K. The communication gap in the ICU: A possible solution. *Nursing Critical Care* 1996, vol. 1, no. 5, pp. 241–4.

Yalom, I. *Love's Executioner.* Bloomsbury, London, 1989.

Index